The Gluten Free Fat Loss Plan

Your guide to losing fat and
getting fit by eating gluten free

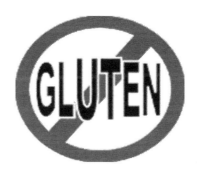

Allison Westfahl

M.S. Exercise Science, NASM-CPT, NASM-PES, USAT

Library of Congress Control Number: 2011907295

Westfahl, Allison.

    The Gluten Free Fat Loss Plan/by Allison Westfahl.

    p.cm

ISBN 978-0-9832554-0-6

Book cover design by Ashley Hoffman; photography by Kirstin Boyer; layout by Amanda Clark of
Grammar Chic, Inc.; editing by Catherine Montrose, Paulina Proper, and Jennifer Wagner.

The information and advice in this book are not meant to replace medical care and consultation. As
with any diet or exercise program, the reader must take full responsibility for his or her own safety and
obtain a doctor's permission before beginning.

Specific mention of authorities, organizations, books, companies, or brands in this book does not imply
endorsement by said entity of the book, nor does it imply endorsement by the author of said entity.
Specific quotes, data, and mention of scientific studies are all referenced in the bibliography section.

For Brian

My husband, my biggest fan, and my best friend

Table of Contents

Meet the Author

Allison Westfahl is a nationally renowned exercise physiologist, endurance sports coach, and media presence. She was raised on a small sheep farm in rural Kansas, and eventually left to attend Yale University. While there, Allison sang for President Clinton's White House Holiday Party, served on a committee for financial aid reform, and ran her first marathon. She graduated magna cum laude with a B.A. in Classical Music, and was inducted into the Phi Beta Kappa society for academic accomplishment.

After college, Allison moved to Boulder, Colorado to pursue her other love - fitness. In 2002, she became a certified personal trainer through the National Academy of Sports Medicine and founded a training and fitness consulting company called The Athletic Edge. Shortly thereafter, she was named the youngest ever Director of Personal Training at Flatiron Athletic Club in Boulder, a health club that was crowned "Best Gym in America" by *Men's Journal* in 2006. In 2008, she was honored with the prestigious Pursuit of Excellence Award, which is given to only two trainers across the nation. Allison now holds a Master of Science degree in Exercise Science, and has been profiled in both *Athletic Business* and *Fitness Business* magazines for her career accomplishments. Allison's additional certifications include Certified Triathlon Coach through USAT, and Performance Enhancement Specialist through NASM.

Allison has taken her knowledge and passion for fitness into the media as well. She has helped choreograph and served as on-screen talent in six fitness DVDs produced by Gaiam, including Bob Greene's (Oprah's trainer) *8 Week Total Body Makeover*. Allison has also written over twenty articles on the topics of health and fitness, and has been quoted in numerous publications, ranging from the *Denver Post* to *Bicycling* magazine to *Shape* magazine.

Allison maintains a busy personal training practice in Colorado, where she works with a wide variety of people, including 15 year old soccer players, 70 year old retirees, and world-class professional athletes. In her spare time, Allison enjoys singing with a professional chamber choir in Denver, playing Trivial Pursuit with her husband Brian, and cooking with too much garlic. Her website is www.allisonwestfahl.com.

Acknowledgements

Writing a book is never the exclusive effort of one individual, and this project was no exception. My sincerest, heartfelt thanks go out to the following people:

To my parents: Mom, you're an extraordinary gluten-free cook, and I've shamelessly stolen many of your best creations over the years. Dad, you are an uncompromising and discriminating judge of gluten-free foods, a skill that you're always happy to put to use.

To all of my friends and family who have not only put up with my commitment to being gluten free, but have welcomed and encouraged it in their own homes by cooking wonderful, delicious gluten-free dishes.

A special thanks goes out to all of my gluten-free clients who are profiled throughout the book. You are wonderful examples of how living gluten free is obtainable, and your willingness to share your stories and your lives is helping to spread the gluten free fat loss message.

To the incredible team of professionals who contributed to this book: Sally Walker, make-up artist; Amy Kender, hair; Kirsten Boyer, photography; Catherine Montrose, Paulina Proper, and Jennifer Wagner, editing; Ashley Hoffman, cover design and website; Amanda Clark, formatting.

Most importantly, to my husband Brian, for being a tireless supporter of this project. Without his relentless encouragement, this book would have remained a wistful idea in the mind of a mildly overactive health fanatic.

PART ONE

The Connection Between Gluten and Fat Loss

Chapter 1

No Gluten Allergy Required-
This Diet is for Everyone!

The Gluten Free Fat Loss Plan is not a fad diet or a get-skinny-quick plan that I created for my personal training clientele. It's a healthy, realistic, and effective method of losing fat and getting fit by cutting out an ingredient that has been sabotaging our waistlines for years: gluten.

As little as 10 years ago, few Americans had ever heard of gluten. Today the *New York Times* regularly publishes gluten-free recipes, the 2010 winning Superbowl quarterback lauded his gluten-free diet in *Sports Illustrated*—even TV personality Elisabeth Hasselbeck has written a book on living gluten-free. Restaurants and food manufacturers are also jumping on the bandwagon: over 80 food manufacturers in the US offer gluten-free products, and 27 national restaurant chains (including P.F. Chang's and Applebee's) now offer gluten-free menus.

But wait, you say! I'm not allergic to gluten, so why should I deprive myself of the wonderful breads, baked goods, and processed foods I love? It is true that most books, cookbooks and websites out there are targeting people who know that they have gluten intolerance, celiac disease, or some other medical reason for eliminating gluten. However, almost every American has at least one health concern that can be linked to gluten, and the biggest concern of all is being fat. The link between eating gluten and being overweight is compelling (see Chapter 3: *Why Gluten is Making You Fat*), yet a diet book addressing this issue does not exist....until now.

As an exercise physiologist, I have worked with thousands of clients who are struggling to lose weight and get fit. Most of them have already run the diet gauntlet by the time they come to see me. Atkins, South Beach, Cabbage Soup - you name it, they've tried it. Most of these diets work initially because they produce rapid weight loss in a short amount of time. But after one, two, three, even eight weeks on the diet, the same harsh reality begins to surface: The Diet is not sustainable. You have a life to live, lunch meetings to attend, family birthday parties to throw - how can you follow a ridiculous protocol of zero carbs and steamed endive boats?!

At the office holiday party, you throw up your hands in frustration and decide to just have a cookie. One cookie can't hurt, right? Then you weigh yourself the next morning and you've gained back THREE POUNDS! How is that even possible? It's because you never really lost the three pounds to begin with - you were simply dehydrated from the lack of carbs in your diet. Each gram of carbohydrate stores four grams of water along with it, so when you cut out carbs you are essentially dehydrating the body on a cellular level. The result is that the number on the scale takes a nosedive, but it's a false victory. You didn't lose fat - you just lost water, and the second you eat something with carbs your body will replenish the missing water and you will "gain" the weight back immediately. I'll bet your low-carb diet books forgot to tell you that.

How this Diet Was Created

In 2004, my mother's sister was diagnosed with celiac disease, a serious autoimmune disorder caused by a complete inability to digest any food containing gluten. My aunt's diagnosis brought the terms "gluten" and "celiac" onto my radar. Concerned that this disease can be hereditary, my mother suggested that I try eating gluten free as a preemptive strike of sorts. I agreed to give it a whirl, but this was *not* easy for a carbophile such as myself. I had essentially lived on pasta, bread, and anything from a bakery my entire life. However, I was curious about celiac because I had some of the symptoms listed on the celiac.org website, so I made a commitment to try gluten-free eating for six months.

The results were powerful. The first and most dramatic difference I noticed was that my severe case of endometriosis all but disappeared. But the benefits didn't stop there: I lost 15 pounds effortlessly, I no longer needed my afternoon nap, and I wasn't bloated and gassy anymore. To top it all off, my athletic performance went through the roof! This was wonderful news for me both personally and professionally. I had just started a career as an exercise physiologist, and my company, The Athletic Edge, was still in its infancy. Could it be that gluten was the secret culprit behind people's struggles with losing weight and getting fit?

I did more research, and discovered several articles linking gluten to food cravings, inability to lose weight, and subpar athletic performance. Eager to test my theory that gluten was a dietary time bomb, I did the only logical thing a young, impetuous personal trainer would do - I asked my entire clientele to start eating gluten free. No blood, urine, or antibody tests were done first. I asked my clients to take measurements and body fat percentages before they started. I also asked everyone to keep detailed food journals that recorded what they ate, how they felt, how they were sleeping, and what their level of satiety was after meals.

Only one client started my gluten-free plan with obvious symptoms of gluten intolerance, and those symptoms disappeared almost immediately when she cut out gluten. The rest of my clients were just like you: overweight, confused, discouraged, and tired of the endless cycle of losing and gaining weight on fad diets. I offered them a delicious, easy-to-follow meal plan that was also gluten free, and inch by inch, waistlines started shrinking and pounds started falling off…for *everyone.*

I was very pleased with the results, but my clients were absolutely ecstatic. More importantly, people were able to lose the weight and keep it off without ever starving or spending days drinking nothing but cayenne-laced water. Though I have had the pleasure of coaching countless clients, family members and friends through my Gluten Free Fat Loss Plan over the years, I have chosen only four of them to profile in this book. These are real people, real before and after pictures, and real stories written in their own words. Now it's your turn to become the next Gluten Free Fat Loss success story!

How to Use This Book

The book is divided into three parts. **Part One: The Connection Between Gluten and Fat Loss** is a detailed explanation of why gluten is a hidden culprit in America's inability to control its waistline. In this section you will learn exactly what gluten is and in what foods it is found. The most extensive chapter in Part One is called "Why Gluten is Making You Fat." If you're tempted to skip any chapters in this book, please make sure it's not this one! In so many diet books, the author asks the reader to "just trust me - it works." To me, this means that either there isn't enough science behind the book's thesis to justify even a small chapter, or the author hasn't done enough research to uncover and explain the science. I'll explain clearly and in detail why eating gluten free assists in fat loss, so you will walk away feeling informed, empowered, and most of all excited about following this diet.

Part Two: Your Gluten Free Fat Loss Meal Plans and Workout Programs are the real nitty gritty of the book. Here you will find sample meal plans as well as an explanation of how you can create your own meals. There are three phases to the Gluten Free Fat Loss Plan:

1. <u>Phase I:</u> Start in this phase if you have more than 10 pounds to lose.
2. <u>Phase II:</u> Move to this phase once you only have 10 pounds left, or start here if you only have 10 pounds total to lose.
3. <u>Phase III:</u> Move to this phase when you have reached your goal weight and want to maintain your fat loss.

Within each of the three phases, there is a meal plan for people who cook and a separate meal plan for people who don't cook. That's right, I've created a fat loss plan that doesn't require countless hours in the kitchen preparing your next meal or snack. My philosophy towards diet and fitness has always been "If it's not realistic, it will never work." If you don't cook, chances are you won't start now, and thanks to the expanding availability of pre-made gluten-free foods, you don't have to! Some of the meals and snacks require assembly, but none of them require more than five minutes of your time.

In Part Two you will also find an extensive exercise section complete with weekly workout programs and pictures demonstrating all the exercises. Losing fat and getting fit does require a commitment to moving your body, but it doesn't have to require an expensive gym membership. My workout program uses only a mat or carpet. I'll show you how to sculpt your muscles, tighten your core, and increase your cardiovascular conditioning by using your body weight as resistance.

Part Three: **The Recipes** contains over thirty of my favorite gluten-free recipes. Each recipe has detailed nutritional information as well as serving sizes, so you can really keep track of your intake. I've also included the "Allowed Food Count" for each recipe. For example, a recipe may say that it contains 1 grey carbohydrate, 1 protein, and 1 other. Take this information and plug it into your daily Nutrition Log so that you can keep track of your allowed foods for the day. Remember, fat loss is all about calories in versus calories out, and tracking your food will help you achieve your fat loss goals quickly and effectively.

Part Four: Appendices, Resources, and References. Here you will find indispensable resources for living a fit, gluten-free life, including lists of well-known restaurants that offer gluten free menus, and websites that offer recipes and advice. I've also gone one step further and earmarked my favorite gluten-free brands for specific foods. When I first started eating gluten free, I spent almost a year wasting my time and money on box after box of inedible pasta and cardboard-like bread. I will not let you suffer the same tribulation!

Jennifer's Gluten Free Fat Loss Story

I'm one of those people for whom switching to a gluten free diet was one of the most profound changes I've ever made.

Three years ago I was clinically obese - 215 pounds and only 5'3" tall. I was also suffering from chronic fatigue, headaches, joint pain, muscle pain, brain fog, and irritable bowel syndrome. I knew that I had to make some radical changes if I wanted to live a happier, healthier lifestyle, and that's when I decided to commit to the Gluten Free Fat Loss Plan. This is my honest feedback: The first two weeks are hard. I quickly learned that in order to feel like I wasn't depriving myself, it was necessary for me to keep all of my favorite rituals. I would meet my best friend for breakfast and just bring along a piece of gluten free bread and have the restaurant toast it. This really helped me establish a new routine and learn that you *can* eat healthy all the time, even when you're going out. I also forced myself to commit to working out regularly. For me, this was just as hard as finally paying attention to what I was eating. I'm not the kind of person who just craves a heavy workout, but the good news is that the plan Allison put together is challenging yet very do-able.

Today I'm strong, healthy, confident, and thrilled to be living gluten free!

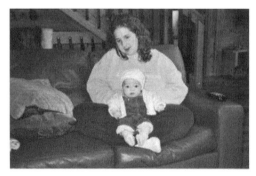

Jennifer at 215 pounds

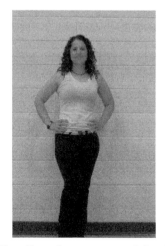

Jennifer at her current weight of
135 pounds

Chapter 2

What is Gluten?

In   recent   years, the term gluten has become a popular dietary buzz word. After all, you're probably reading this book because you keep seeing words like gluten, gluten-free, gluten intolerance, gluten sensitivity, and you've said to yourself, "I'm curious about all this gluten stuff, but um....I don't even know what gluten is!"

Here is the textbook definition of gluten:

> *Gluten is a binding protein found in wheat, barley and rye. More specifically, it's two proteins called gliadin and glutenin. These proteins are found in the endosperm of the aforementioned grass-related grains.*

If you think this definition is convoluted and unclear, you're right. It's no wonder we're all so confused about gluten - it's a protein, it's actually two proteins, it's only found in part of the grain, it's in more than one grain, it's in some grains but not others......and the confusion doesn't stop there. Gluten can be found in maize (corn) and rice as well, but this type of gluten lacks the gliadin molecule, so it's not classified as a "true gluten" and does not contribute to the symptoms seen with gluten intolerance. The real problem, then, is the combination of glutenin and gliadin. However, "gliadin and glutenin free" doesn't exactly roll off the tongue, so I can see why "gluten free" won the nomenclature contest.

Of the three gluten-containing grains, wheat has the highest amount of gluten, and coincidentally it's also the grain that Americans consume the most. In particular, we consume lots of wheat endosperms because it's the largest part of a kernel of grain (approximately 83 percent of the kernel weight). Of further interest is the fact that the endosperm also contains the highest concentration of gluten. Keep this factoid in mind as you read the definitions of whole, refined, and enriched grains in Chapter 3. For now, let's take a look at a kernel of wheat to get a better understanding of where gluten comes from.

A Kernel of Wheat

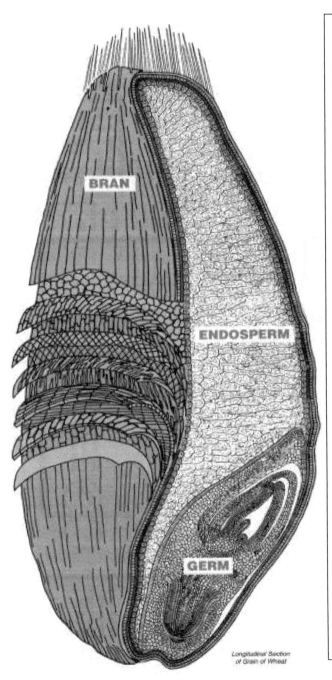

Longitudinal Section
of Grain of Wheat

The Wheat Kernel

…sometimes called the wheat berry, the kernel is the seed from which the wheat plant grows. Each tiny seed contains three distinct parts that are separated during the milling process to produce flour.

Endosperm

…about 83 percent of the kernel weight, and the source of white flour. The endosperm contains the greatest share of protein, carbohydrates and iron, as well as the major B-vitamins, such as riboflavin, niacin, and thiamine. It is also a source of soluble fiber.

Bran

…about 14 ½ percent of the kernel weight. Bran is included in whole wheat flour, and can also be bought separately. The bran contains a small amount of protein, large quantities of the B-vitamins, trace minerals, and dietary fiber – primarily soluble.

Germ

…about 2 ½ percent of the kernel weight. The germ is the embryo or sprouting section of the seed, often separated from flour in milling because the fat content (10 percent) limits shelf life. The germ contains minimal quantities of high quality protein and a greater share of B-complex vitamins and trace minerals. Wheat germ can be purchased separately and is part of whole wheat flour.

- *Reprinted with permission from The Wheat Foods Council, www.wheatfoods.org*

Now you know what gluten is and in which grains it can be found, but what about the foods and derivatives that are made from these grains? Because wheat, barley, and rye are so versatile, they show up in lots of places that don't seem obvious.

Thanks to the *Food Allergen Labeling and Consumer Protection Act of 2004**, food manufacturers in the United States are required by law to identify wheat and wheat derivatives very clearly on the list of ingredients. Unfortunately, the other two gluten-containing grains (rye and barley) aren't considered a "major allergen," so as a consumer you still need to learn how to identify barley, rye, and hidden sources of wheat in foods you eat.

When you embark on a gluten-free diet, realize that just because a food is labeled "Wheat Free" does not mean that it is also "Gluten Free." If a product is labeled wheat free, it may still contain rye or barley, and both of those grains contain gluten. Still confused? Think of a big bowl of fruit. In that bowl there are three different types of fruits: apples, oranges, and pears. All three of these items in the bowl are fruits, but they aren't all oranges. The same is true of gluten. Wheat, barley, and rye all fall under the larger category of gluten-containing grains, but only one is wheat. This is why you must be extremely diligent about reading your food labels and checking for gluten derivatives even if the product says that it is Wheat Free.

Look at the following list of gluten-containing foods and you will realize just how pervasive it is in the American Diet.

*To view the complete document, visit www.fda.gov/Food/LabelingNutrition/FoodAllergensLabeling

Gluten-containing Grains:

- Wheat
- Barley
- Rye

Foods That Contain Gluten:
(Unless the food is specifically labeled "Gluten Free")

- Bagels
- Barley, Barley grass, Barley Malt
- Beer
- Biscuits
- Bran
- Bread (even sourdough and potato bread)
- Bread crumbs
- Breading of any kind, including tempura
- Brewer's yeast

- Bulgur Wheat, Bulgur Nuts
- Cake (including all cake mixes)
- Candy (check label)
- Cereal
- Chilton
- Chow Mein Noodles
- Croissants and all pastries
- Cookies (including oatmeal cookies)
- Couscous
- Crackers, Melba Toast
- Croutons
- Doughnuts
- Dumplings
- Durum and Durum flour (this is a type of wheat)
- Flour tortillas (including low carb varieties)
- Fried foods
- Germ (i.e. wheat germ)
- Graham flour
- Gravy
- Groats
- Hydrolyzed vegetable protein
- Ice cream cones
- Kamut
- Kasha (when made from wheat, barley, or rye)
- Macaroni
- Malt, malt extract, malt syrup, malt flavoring, malt vinegar
- Matzo meal, Matzo soup, Matzo balls
- Miso soup
- Monosodium glutamate (MSG)
- Muffins
- Noodles
- Pancakes and waffles
- Pasta
- Pearl barley
- Pies
- Pizza crust
- Popovers, Pop Tarts
- Pretzels
- Rolls

- Rye (including rye bread)
- Seitan
- Semolina, semolina triticum
- Shoyu
- Soba noodles
- Soy sauce
- Sprouted wheat (brands like Ezekiel are not gluten free)
- Stuffing
- Tabbouleh
- Teriyaki sauce
- Textured Vegetable Protein
- Triticale
- Udon (including Udon noodles)
- Wheat and anything that contains the word "wheat"

Foods That Sometimes Contain Gluten:

And you thought we were done?! The following foods sometimes use gluten or gluten derivatives as fillers or thickeners. This is when you truly have to become a food detective. Remember, the Food Labeling Act of 2004 does not require that gluten derivatives be identified on labels, so it is up to you to be educated about what your food truly contains. Here are some of the main culprits that sometimes contain gluten:

- Alcoholic beverages
- Baking powder
- Beverage mixes (i.e. instant chocolate drinks and some diet shake mixes)
- Blue cheese (sometimes made with bread)
- Bouillon Cubes and Broth
- Canned baked beans
- Caramel color (including sodas and diet sodas)
- Chocolate syrup
- Cold cuts
- Custard
- Chorizo
- Creamers (especially the flavored ones)
- Frozen dinners
- Fruit fillings
- Ground spices
- Hot dogs

- Ice cream
- Imitation fish (imitation crab meat and lobster often contain wheat)
- Instant oats and instant oatmeal
- Ketchup
- Marshmallows and marshmallow crème
- Potato chips (i.e. Sun Chips and other whole grain chips)
- Pudding
- Root beer
- Salad dressings
- Sauces (be careful when ordering in restaurants)
- Sausages
- Stabilizers
- Steak sauce

Foods That Do Not Contain Gluten:

You almost stopped reading after that long list of no-nos, didn't you? The good news is that the list of foods that are naturally gluten free is even longer than the list of foods that do contain gluten. Please keep in mind that the following list refers only to foods in their natural, whole state. As you can tell from the list of gluten-containing foods above, any naturally gluten-free food can quickly enter the no-no list if it is cooked or prepared with gluten ingredients. And herein lies the rub about the typical American diet: We have strayed from eating foods in their natural, whole state. Instead, our diets consist of highly prepared, processed, and packaged foods. Eat the following foods in their natural state and you will also be naturally gluten free:

- All vegetables, including starchy vegetables such as potatoes, yams, squash, beets
- All fruits
- All meat, poultry, fish
- All beans (dried and canned), legumes, tofu (only in its natural state, not texturized vegetable protein)
- Most dairy products (beware of blue cheese and flavored ice creams and yogurts)
- All nuts and nut butters (beware of flavored nut butters and nuts roasted with soy sauce)
- Cider vinegar, wine vinegar, distilled vinegar
- Fresh herbs, cream of tartar, baking soda, sugar
- Tea, coffee
- Sugar, most jams, honey, agave nectar

Here is the exciting part...the following grains and flours are also gluten free:

- Almond flour
- Amaranth
- Arrowroot
- Bean flour
- Besan
- Brown rice, white rice, and brown and white rice flours
- Buckwheat
- Cassava
- Corn flour, Corn meal, Corn starch
- Cottonseed
- Dal
- Flaxseed
- Job's tears
- Manioc
- Millet
- Milo
- Pea flour
- Polenta, Polenta flour
- Potato flour
- Quinoa
- Sago
- Soy flour
- Tapioca flour
- Taro flour
- Teff
- Yucca

I will explain in detail how to incorporate these yummy gluten-free foods into your new fat loss plan in Part Two. As you can see already, you'll be eating lots of fruits and veggies, lean protein, healthy fats, and some new grains you probably haven't tried before. It would be a good idea to print out pages 23-27 and keep them nearby until you feel you have a handle on exactly which food items contain gluten. As with any new regimen, there is a learning curve; however, I guarantee that in a few short weeks you'll be able to spot gluten a mile away!

Chapter 3

Why Gluten is Making You Fat

As previously mentioned, Americans absolutely love to eat gluten, particularly wheat products. The United States is the third largest producer of wheat in the world, which makes wheat affordable, available, and convenient for us as consumers. In 2010, the United States produced 2.2 billion bushels of wheat, and we snarfed it up at the alarming rate of 137 pounds per capita (per person per year). Unfortunately, most of the wheat we consume looks nothing like those amber waves of grain by the time it actually reaches our plate.

In its original form, wheat is a good source of manganese, fiber, and the amino acids cystine and tryptophan. However, as our consumption of processed foods, fast foods, and "Frankenfoods" continues to rise, those nutritional benefits are quickly stripped away. In fact, our previous notion of wheat as a "superfood" may be incorrect. Jonny Bowden, author of *The 150 Healthiest Foods on Earth,* argues that "grains have a host of nutritional shortcomings. It's finally becoming accepted wisdom that the refined grains - which constitute most of our cereals, pastas, and breads - are absolutely useless nutritionally."

They may be useless, but oh man, do they taste good! Yes, yes they do. But a moment on the lip, a lifetime on…the blood glucose, the arteries, and the waistline. Gluten-containing foods are secretly sabotaging our health in four ways:

1. Gluten-containing foods are often made from highly processed and refined grains
2. Most gluten-containing foods are calorie rich and nutrient poor
3. Gluten-containing foods are frequently high in refined sugar
4. Gluten-containing foods can trigger bingeing and food addiction

1. Gluten-containing foods are often made from highly processed and refined grains

Do you truly know what percentage of your daily grain intake is in whole form? The USDA recommends that we consume a total of 6.30 ounces of grains per day, half of which should come from whole grain sources. This means you should eat three servings of whole grains a day. This shouldn't be too difficult, considering that one serving is ½ cup of cooked brown rice, ½ cup of cooked whole grain pasta, or one slice of whole grain bread.

Unfortunately, we are not making those choices. According to a 2007 study by the USDA, only 7% of Americans are getting the recommended daily dose of whole grains. Yet Americans are consuming *more total* grains than recommended; on average we eat 6.68 ounces of grains per day, and 5.61 of those ounces are refined. Many of you may be smirking right now and thinking that you're one of the 7% of Americans who actually get their whole grains. After all, you order wheat bread at restaurants, you buy pasta that says "whole grain", and you get the multi-grain bagel at the coffee shop in the morning. Ha ha, you say! I'm eating healthy!

Not so fast, my friend. That wheat bread at the restaurant contains refined wheat flour, not whole wheat. Whole grain pasta may only contain 1% whole grain, while the other 99% is refined. And finally, your multi-grain bagel is most likely made from three different types (multi) of *refined* grains. If you feel tricked and confused by food labeling, you should. The underlying problem is that food manufacturers use healthy-sounding terms, knowing that consumers won't do their homework to figure out what those terms really mean. Well, get ready to become an informed consumer. Here is a crash course into frequently-used grain terminology. Refer to the diagram on page 22 for a reminder of the different parts of a kernel of wheat.

Whole grains:
Whole grains shall consist of the intact, ground, cracked or flaked caryopsis, whose principal anatomical components - the starchy endosperm, germ and bran - are present in the same relative proportions as they exist in the intact caryopsis.

Refined grains:
Grains that have been modified or refined from their original composition by removing the bran and germ. Refining techniques frequently include mixing, bleaching, and bromating.

Enriched grains:
Grains that have been refined (bran and germ removed) and stripped of key nutrients such as fiber, iron, and folic acid. After processing, these nutrients are added back in, thereby enriching the grain. Many times the nutrients that are added back are not in the same form; for example, metallic iron can be used. Furthermore, added nutrients commonly represent a fraction of what the original grain contained.

Fortified grains:
Essentially the same as enriched grains, except that fortified grains have nutrients added to them that never originally existed in the grain, as opposed to nutrients that once existed but were removed.

These definitions clearly show why whole grains are more nutritionally sound than refined grains, but they don't really explain why refined grains contribute to unwanted body weight. This is why: stripping the bran and germ from the grain also strips the fiber away, which in turn causes the body to digest the grain quickly and also makes insulin spike. If your body is digesting food quickly, then you are prone to eat more calories than necessary because you don't feel full. As a reaction to all these extra calories, your body releases too much insulin and your blood sugar starts to take a roller coaster ride. Scientists at the Harvard School for Public Health agree, stating that "easily digested refined carbohydrates …may contribute to weight gain, interfere with weight loss, and promote diabetes and heart disease."

In Part Two of this book, I will explain in detail how to make sure the gluten-free grains you are eating on the diet are also whole grain. The last thing you want is to trade in your refined gluten-containing grains for refined gluten-free grains.

2. Most gluten-containing foods are calorically rich and nutrient poor

Despite the fact that many wheat-based foods are extremely high in calories and low in nutritive value, Americans insist on consuming them on a regular basis. Consider the following statistics:

*In any given month, approximately 93% of Americans eat at least one pizza.

*Almost 50% of Americans eat cereal for breakfast. The top 10 most popular cereals in the United States are: *General Mills' Cheerios, Kellogg's Special K, Post's Honey Bunches of Oats, Kellogg's Frosted Flakes, Kellogg's Frosted Mini Wheats, Kellogg's Raisin Bran, Kellogg's Froot Loops, General Mills' Cinnamon Toast Crunch, General Mills' Lucky Charms, and Quaker Oats' Cap'n Crunch.* **The average sugar content per serving in each of these cereals is more than that of a jelly doughnut.**

*A *Chipotle* chicken burrito (made with a large flour tortilla) with rice, black beans, and cheese contains 830 calories (over half my daily recommendation for weight loss), 28 grams of fat (11 grams of which are saturated), and 1,620 mg of sodium (almost 70% the RDA).

Other popular gluten-containing foods in the American diet are bagels, donuts, muffins, cookies, bread, buns, and a whole host of snack foods including pretzels, granola, and energy bars. All these foods are high in refined grains, high in added sugar, and low in fiber and nutrients. It's no surprise that foods like pizza and donuts are not healthy choices, but granola and pretzels are also very unhealthy. I'm not sure how granola came to be viewed as a health food, but the binding ingredient that holds all those healthy oats together is sugar, and the dried fruits that make that same granola taste so yummy are mainly just, well, sugar. To add insult to injury, granola is extremely high in calories - a typical serving of ¼ cup is well over 250 calories. If you're in the habit of filling a cereal bowl to the brim with granola and then topping it off with skim milk, you're packing in about 1,000 calories and well over 50 grams of sugar. The bottom line is that all those beloved breads, cereals, and snack foods that you thought were so healthy can be nutritional suicide.

3. Gluten-containing foods are frequently high in refined sugar

Let's start with the usual suspect: bread. Take a stroll through the bakery section at your local grocery store and see how many loaves of bread you can find that do not contain an ingredient ending in "ose." Anything ending in "ose" falls into the category of a sugar. Some frequent names that show up on ingredient lists are fructose, lactose, maltose, and sucrose (white sugar). Of course, sugar itself is frequently listed as an ingredient, along with corn syrup (high fructose corn syrup), brown sugar, and honey.

Most "ose" ingredients are located second in the product list, which means that some form of sugar is second only to wheat (usually refined, as you know now) in bread ingredients by volume. Hmmm, sounds pretty nutritionally poor to me. In fact, adding sugar to bread products has become the go-to method for increasing sales and consumer loyalty. After all, sugar makes products taste better, and if a boring old piece of wheat bread tastes like honey, then hey - sign me up for that!

According to the USDA, added sugar consumption amongst Americans is currently at the astounding rate of 156 pounds per capita. That's *added* sugar, which does not include naturally occurring sugar such as that found in fruit. Just how much is 156 pounds of sugar? It is 67,704 grams or 16,068 teaspoons. This is how much every American averages *per year!* It almost seems physically impossible that a human being could consume that much; every item of food we eat would have to be laden with added sugar. In fact, it is. Much like the whole grain debacle, food manufacturers use clever wording to disguise the amount of sugar contained in the products we eat.

A perfect example is Starbucks' attempt to offer healthier breakfast options such as the Low-fat Red Raspberry Breakfast Muffin. At first glance, this may seem like a good choice. The product is labeled as "low-fat" and it contains fruit, two qualities which sound very healthy. Now take a closer look at the both the nutritional content and the ingredient list and you'll be shocked to discover the unhealthy nature of this muffin:

Starbucks Low-fat Red Raspberry Muffin
Total serving size:128 grams
Total calories per serving: 340
Total fat: 6 grams
Total carbohydrates: 65 grams
Total sugar: 37 grams
Total protein: 7 grams

Ingredient list:
unbleached, enriched wheat flour (wheat flour, malted barley flour, niacin, reduced iron, thiamine mononitrate, riboflavin, folic acid), sugar, raspberries, buttermilk (cultured pasteurized nonfat milk, salt, sodium citrate), water, whole eggs, nonfat yogurt (cultured pasteurized nonfat milk, inulin, pectin, active cultures), lemon peel, soybean oil, orange juice concentrate, nonfat milk powder, baking powder (sodium acid pyrophosphate, sodium bicarbonate, cornstarch, monocalcium phosphate), invert sugar, salt, unsalted butter (cream [from milk]), natural flavor, konjac gum.

When evaluating the nutritional benefits of a food item, it's important to consider the mathematical breakdown of its component parts. This muffin has a total weight of 128 grams. 65 grams come from carbohydrates, meaning that 51% of the muffin is carbs. Now look at the ingredient list - not a single one of those carbs comes from a whole grain source. Instead, the carbohydrates come from unbleached, enriched flour (i.e. NOT whole grain) and a host of sugar-containing ingredients. Speaking of sugar, this muffin has a whopping 37 grams, which constitutes 29% of the total muffin. 37 grams of sugar is equal to 9.25 teaspoons, or 3.25 grams over the FDA's recommended daily intake of 6 teaspoons. The overall score card of this supposedly healthy breakfast option? D+ at best.

I challenge you to spend a day adding up the grams of sugar that are in your food. Yes, this means you will have to read labels and do some research, but hey - not paying attention to what goes into your mouth is how you gained weight in the first place. If you want to reverse the expansion of your belly, then you'd better start paying attention to your sugar intake. Remember that the FDA says you should be consuming no more than 6 teaspoons, or 24 grams, of added sugar per day. That 12 ounce Dr. Pepper that you just had for lunch contains 41 grams. Yikes. And now you start to see how consuming 16,068 teaspoons of sugar per year is possible.

I believe you should be eating no more than 50 grams of sugar per day *including* naturally-occurring sugars that are found in fruits, vegetables, and dairy products. I go into great detail about which foods are highest in sugar in the meal plan section of the book. Besides being gluten free, the other main focus of this diet is to drastically cut down the amount of sugar you eat and eliminate your addiction to sweets.

4. Gluten-containing foods can trigger bingeing and food addiction

You might be looking at statement #4 right now and thinking, "Ok, now she's gone too far. I was with her for the whole sugar/refined grain/calorie dense part, but this?" I'm going to defend my position by giving you yet another homework assignment: Think back to the last five times you overate (binged) and list the foods you binged on. Let me guess - they all contain gluten, right? The only exceptions may be ice cream and chocolate, but even many of those products contain hidden gluten. Part two of your homework assignment: Write down the foods that you truly feel you can't live without, or that you feel would be *extremely* difficult to cut out of your diet. My guess is that a pattern is starting to emerge in your two lists. You're writing down the same foods over and over: breads, bagels, muffins, cookies, and donuts - all products that contain gluten. If you have often felt that baked goods are literally holding you hostage and forcing you to make poor food choices, you're not alone, and you're not crazy.

Those feelings are a reaction to substances called exorphins, which are found in gluten and have been shown to have narcotic-like effects. Narcotics produce an initial "high" that causes feelings of mild euphoria, which is quickly followed by tiredness, moodiness, regret....and then a desire to go back for more. In other words, gluten can act like a drug in the body, and if you're addicted to a drug, then you will experience horrible withdrawal symptoms if you don't have it regularly.

I'd like to share a real-life example of this phenomenon from a client of mine. Her story may sound very familiar to what you're experiencing in your own struggles with weight loss. Jan (name changed for privacy) came to me in 2007 in a state of desperation; she had tried every diet plan on the market, she was working out two hours a day, and she was increasingly disgusted by the size of her stomach.

I asked Jan to keep a food journal to reveal her current eating habits. A few things immediately jumped out at me. First, she was living on low-carb bread, low-carb tortillas, low-carb pretzels, low-carb everything. Second, she had a habit of munching on granola as a "healthy" snack in the afternoons. Although Jan thought she was eating healthy, she was actually ingesting high amounts of both gluten and sugar. As soon as I switched her to a gluten-free diet, she immediately lost the stubborn pounds, and most of them came off her belly. Additionally, she completely lost her cravings for carbs and sugary foods, and she felt in control of her food choices for the first time in her life.

Because the study of gluten is relatively new, being able to provide irrefutable, time-tested evidence that gluten foods can be addictive and contribute to weight gain is a little like trying to paint the wind. However, as more experts take on the study of gluten, one of the emerging conclusions is that omitting gluten from your diet is a sure-fire path to feeling and looking better. Dr. Stephen Wangen, author of *Healthier without Wheat: A New Understanding of Wheat Allergies, Celiac Disease, and Non-Celiac Gluten Intolerance*, says:

> Research, as well as feedback from patients, has shown that a tremendous number of problems can be triggered by a gluten intolerance. Many people actually have symptoms completely opposite of what we used to think defined gluten intolerance - they suffer from constipation and weight gain triggered by gluten. In fact, many celiacs are overweight when they are diagnosed with celiac disease.

It's time for you to get rid of that unwanted weight and bloat by voting gluten off the diet island! Are you on board? Are you ready to take control of your health, your diet, and your bulging belly? If you're nervously biting your nails and tentatively shaking your head yes right now, I want you to think about this: whatever you have tried in the past clearly didn't work. If it had, you wouldn't be reading this book. We've all heard this adage a million times but I'm going to say it once more…..the definition of insanity is someone who continues to do the same thing over and over again and expects different results. Stop running around on your dietary hamster wheel and jump off into the world of gluten-free-dom!

Troy's Gluten Free Fat Loss Story

As an avid cyclist, I consumed a large amount of gluten products for years. Then last year my wife was diagnosed with a severe allergy to both gluten and dairy, so I decided to cut it out of my diet as well in order to be supportive. I couldn't believe the difference it made! As you can see from the photos, my gut pretty much disappeared, and my desire to ride my bike has increased drastically as well as my ability to ride for a long time. I no longer feel like I'm "crashing" in the middle of a ride, nor do I bonk when I get home. I've also noticed that my mental sharpness is much better - I'm able to ride at a higher level of intensity with less fear because my thinking feels more acute. My trick is to eat some healthy complex carbs before I exercise, then some lean protein and avocado afterwards for optimal muscle recovery.

One final thing: my wife and I live in France, so if we can happily live a gluten and dairy free life in this land full of bread and cheese, then there is no excuse for you!

After

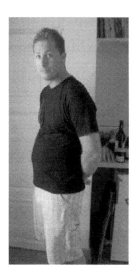

Before

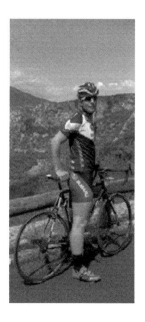

Chapter 4

Additional Health Benefits of Eating Gluten Free

Losing weight and getting fit is reason enough to eat gluten free, but for many of you the benefits will just *start* there. Maybe you chose this book because you've been wondering if you have gluten intolerance, and you figured that losing a few pounds in the process would be a handy double-whammy. You're not alone. Recent statistics estimate that 1 in 32 Americans suffer from a diagnosed form of gluten intolerance. In addition, countless cases of gluten intolerance are "silent," undiagnosed and untreated for years, sometimes even for a lifetime. Gluten intolerance often goes undetected because many of its symptoms aren't obviously connected to diet.

Symptoms of Gluten Intolerance:

- Abdominal pain
- Anemia
- Bloating
- Chronic fatigue
- Constipation
- Cramping
- Depression
- Diarrhea
- Endometriosis
- Fibromyalgia
- Frequent infections: eyes, sinuses, mouth, vagina, respiratory, digestive tract, urinary tract
- Infertility
- Irritable bowel syndrome
- Mood swings
- Osteoporosis
- Unexplained weight gain
- Unexplained weight loss

This list is a smorgasbord of mild to severe health conditions that could affect anyone at any time. To further complicate the situation, these symptoms can be erratic and inconsistent. One day, eating a slice of wheat bread makes you horribly gassy and constipated; the next day it has no effect at all. I've watched clients fall on and off the gluten-free wagon for years because one day they accidentally ate something with gluten and felt fine, which then snow-balled into "oh look, I don't have an intolerance anymore," so they went back to a gluten-filled diet. Inevitably, over the next few weeks, their original symptoms start to reappear. They acknowledge that gluten is once again a problem, and jump back on the gluten-free wagon.

Gluten intolerance, by any other name, would be just as . . .

confusing. Terminology in the world of gluten intolerance can be very complicated, and it's helpful to have a decoder ring to help clear up the muddiness. Here is a short list of terms that all refer to gluten intolerance in one form or another:

Gluten intolerance, gluten sensitivity, celiac sprue, celiac disease, non-celiac gluten intolerance, gluten sensitive enteropathy, nontropical sprue. Ugg, my brain hurts. The good news is that all of these terms can be loosely (again, there are plenty of reasons to argue the minutia here) categorized into two camps.

Camp I: gluten intolerance, gluten sensitivity, non-celiac gluten intolerance.

Camp II: celiac sprue, celiac disease, gluten sensitive enteropathy, nontropical sprue.

The terms from Camp I and Camp II are often used interchangeably, which would imply that anyone who has gluten intolerance (Camp I) also has celiac sprue (Camp II). This is not true. Do you remember the fruit analogy from Chapter Two? The same situation applies here: There is a big bowl of fruit called gluten intolerance (Camp I) and within that bowl are countless different types of intolerances, but only one of them is celiac (Camp II).

You can see why so many people - including doctors - assume that gluten intolerance and celiac disease are the same thing, when in fact celiac disease is only one of many different types of gluten intolerance. If you go to your doctor and ask to be tested for celiac disease, your test may come back negative. This does not, however, mean that you can tolerate gluten. In fact, celiac disease affects only 1 in 133 Americans, so the chances are slim that you will test positive for it. Which brings me to another discussion point…

Testing for gluten intolerance

I can pretty much guarantee that cutting out gluten will make you feel better, but some of you will still want to have an irrefutable "positive" result so that you feel confident in your decision to cut out gluten. Unfortunately, because of its finicky nature and sub-clinical symptoms, testing and diagnosing gluten intolerance can be very problematic. Furthermore, because there are countless types of gluten intolerance, no single test can screen for all of them, meaning that you are more likely to test negative than positive. Here are the most common types of tests conducted for gluten intolerance, and the problems with each of them:

Test	Procedure	Problems
Allergy test (skin prick test)	Gliadin is scratched into the skin and then checked for a reaction.	Patient's reaction must be fairly severe for the scratch test to come back positive. Mild reactions are often dismissed.
Antibody blood panel test	Blood is drawn to look for the presence of antibodies to gliadin.	If your results are in the low or low-normal range then the result will be negative, even though most times if people have *any* antibodies present this indicates an intolerance to gluten.
Intestinal biopsy	A small scope is inserted into the small intestine to look for "villous atrophy".	Only reveals celiac sprue, not other forms of intolerance. Furthermore, the patient must present with severe celiac in order for the biopsy to come back positive.
Elimination diet	Follow a gluten-free diet for a period of 30-60 days to determine if your symptoms decrease or disappear.	None!

The allergy test, blood panel test, and intestinal biopsy often produce false negatives because mild or sub-clinical cases go undetected. In order to produce a positive test result, your symptoms must be so far advanced that you may have been suffering for years.

I tested negative on both a blood panel and skin prick test, yet the symptoms I experience when I eat gluten are quite severe: painful bloating and gas, headaches, insomnia, and irritability. Also, I have a family history of celiac disease, so I'm not going to roll the dice and spend the next two decades eating gluten, all the while silently destroying my precious intestinal villi. Eating gluten free is my insurance policy for good health. I hope it becomes yours as well!

PART TWO

Your Gluten Free Fat Loss Meal Plans and Workout Programs

Chapter 5

Getting Started with Your Fat Loss Plan

You finally made it to the actual diet part of the book! This is where I outline exactly which foods are allowed on the diet, how much of them you can have, and how to make sure you are eating them in the right amounts to optimize fat loss. There are three phases to the diet, and most of you will be starting in Phase I. However, if you have ten pounds or less to lose then you can skip immediately to Phase II and start there.

Phase I:
>   This phase is appropriate for anyone who has more than 10 pounds to lose. It's based on a daily caloric intake of 1,400-1,500 calories, which is low enough to stimulate immediate weight loss but not so low that you will be hungry.

Phase II:
>   Phase II is meant to take off those last 10 pounds. This plan is based on 1,500-1,600 calories a day, which will serve as fuel for your increased activity level (you *are* following the workout plan, right?) while still allowing the body to lose pounds and fat.

Phase III:
>   Congrats - you made it! Phase III is a maintenance program that allows you to hold onto your goal weight. It is based on 1,600-1,800 calories a day, and it's a healthy, sustainable way to continue living gluten free while being active.

Basics of the Diet

It will come as no great shock that the main tenet of the diet is to cut out all foods that contain gluten. But that's really just the first step towards creating a healthy, delicious fat loss program. The diet also follows these parameters:

- **No more than 50 total grams of sugar per day, including naturally occurring sugars found in vegetables, fruits, and dairy.**
- **No less than 20 grams of fiber per day.**

- More than half your grains must come from whole grain sources.
- The meal plans follow a ratio of 45%-50% carbohydrates, 25%-30% fats, and 20%-25% protein.
- Eat three meals and two snacks per day.
- Never go longer than 4 hours without eating.
- Drink a minimum of 60 ounces of water per day.

If this sounds like a lot of things to keep track of, don't worry! I've created an easy-to-use system of tracking your foods that is color-coded and divided into different types of foods. All you have to do is look at the number of servings from each group that is allowed each day, check them off on the nutrition logs provided for each phase, and by the end of the day you will have magically eaten a perfectly balanced, delicious diet that will stimulate fat loss.

If this tracking system seems unappealing to you, simply follow the sample meal plans I've created. Isn't this easy? Another advantage to following the meal plans is that you don't have to think about what to eat for your next meal. No stress, no thinking, no problem. In addition to being delicious and easy, the meal plans take into account the cost of a specialized diet. When you first make the switch to eating gluten free, you may find that some items are more expensive than their gluten-containing cousins. That's why I've tailored the meal plans to utilize fresh ingredients before they go bad (e.g. using fresh blueberries in muffins one day, and in a snack the next day) and I've also reduced wasted leftovers from dinner by including them as lunch the next day.

Daily Allowances of Each Food Group

Food Groups	Phase I	Phase II	Phase III
Vegetables	Unlimited, with a minimum of 5 (1 from grey category)	Unlimited, with a minimum of 5 (2 from grey category)	Unlimited, with a minimum of 5 (2 from grey category)
Fruits	2 a day (1 from grey category)	3 a day (1 from grey category)	3 a day (2 from grey category)
Proteins	3 a day (1 from grey category)	4 a day (1 from grey category)	4 a day (2 from grey category)
Grains/Carbs	3 a day (1 from grey category)	3 a day (2 from grey category)	4 a day (2 from grey category)
Fats	2 a day	2 a day	3 a day
Other Foods	2 a day	3 a day	4 a day
Cheat Foods	1 a week	2 a week	3 a week

On the next few pages is a detailed list of foods that are allowed in each category. Some Fruits, Vegetables, Proteins, and Carbohydrates have been shaded in grey. These are the items that are restricted according to the chart on page 44 and will be discussed as being in the "grey category." The Fats, Other Foods, and Cheat Foods don't have grey categories, but please still follow the total number of servings allowed per day in each category.

Vegetables

Vegetables	Serving Size
Alfalfa sprouts, Artichoke, Arugula, Asparagus, Bell pepper (all colors), Bok choy, Broccoli, Brussels sprouts, Cabbage, Cauliflower, Celery, Collard greens, Cucumber, Eggplant, Escarole, Fennel, Green beans, Green cabbage, Green onion, Iceburg lettuce, Jicama, Kale, Leaf lettuce, Mushrooms, Peas, Radish, Snow peas, Spinach, Squash (all varieties), Swiss chard, Tomato	Unlimited!
Grey Category Vegetables	**Serving Size**
Beets, Carrots, Onions, Parsnips, Potatoes, Sweet corn, Sweet potatoes	1 medium sized vegetable (i.e. 1 medium carrot=1 serving)
Peas	1 cup

Fruits

Fruits	Serving Size
Blackberries, Blueberries, Papaya, Raspberries	1 cup
Cantaloupe	¼ of medium
Grapefruit	½ of medium
Honeydew Melon	$^1/_{10}$ of medium
Apricot, Kiwifruit, Plum	2 medium
Lemon, Lime, Nectarine, Orange, Peach, Tangerine	1 medium
Pineapple	½ cup chopped
Strawberries	8 medium
Grey Category Fruits	**Serving Size**
Apple	1 large
Banana, Pear	1 medium
Date	1 large medjool
Grapes	¾ cup
Mango	1 cup sliced
Sweet cherries	21 medium
Watermelon	2 cups diced

Protein

Proteins	Serving Size
Bison, Elk, Rabbit, Venison	4 oz
Ham (*deli meat*)* Chicken and Turkey (*white meat only, deli meat or breasts*)* Extra lean beef (*any cut that is 96% lean or leaner*)	3 oz
Arctic Char, Cod, Crab (*not imitation*), Halibut, Lobster, Pollock, Scallops, Shrimp, Tilapia, Tuna	3 oz
Egg whites	4 whites
Almond cheese	3 oz
Protein powder (*whey or egg white*)*	1 scoop
Greek yogurt (*non-fat, plain, no flavorings*)*	1 cup
Tofu (*extra firm*)	¼ block
Grey Category Proteins	**Serving Size**
Bacon (*pork or turkey, no added sugar, uncured*)	2 small slices
Beef (*any cut that is between 90%-95% lean*)	3 oz
Pork chops, Pork tenderloin	4 oz
Salmon, Trout	3 oz
Oysters	6 oz
Whole eggs	1
Other dark meat sources of protein that contain more than 5 grams of fat	3 oz

*Please read the explanation of allowed proteins on page 50 for details.

It is my strong opinion that you should strive to eat locally-raised, grass-fed sources of protein. Your local farmer's market is always a good resource for these items, as is the website: www.eatwild.com.

Carbohydrate

Carbohydrates	Serving Size
Amaranth*, Buckwheat*, Millet*, Polenta*, Quinoa*, White Rice, Wild Rice*	1 cup cooked
Brown Rice*, Teff*	½ cup cooked
Oatmeal*	1 ¼ cup cooked
Taro root	$^2/_3$ cup cooked
Beans (*all varieties*)	½ cup cooked
Corn tortillas, hard	2 shells
Corn tortillas, soft	3 tortillas
Popcorn* (all natural, nothing added, air popped only)	3 cups popped
Grey Category Carbohydrates	**Serving Size**
Bagel (*gluten-free, whole grain*)	1 small (no more than 300 calories)
Bread (*gluten-free, whole grain*)	2 slices (no more than 100 calories per slice)
Pancakes and waffles (*gluten-free, whole grain*)	2 small (4" diameter)
Rice crackers (*whole grain*)	14 crackers
Rice cakes (*whole grain*)	3 cakes

*These are whole grains unless identified as *enriched, refined, or fortified*. Be sure to check pre-made or boxed varieties of these foods for added gluten ingredients.

Fats

Fats	Serving Size
Avocado	½ of medium
Almonds, Cashews, Hazelnuts, Macadamia nuts, Peanuts, Pecans, Pine nuts, Pistachios	1 oz ($^1/_8$ cup)
Sunflower seeds	2 oz ($^1/_4$ cup)
Almond butter, Cashew butter, Peanut butter, Tahini	1 tbsp
Olives (*green or black*)	15 large or 20 small
Olive oil	1 tbsp

Other Foods

Food	Serving Size
Agave nectar	1 tbsp
Almond milk (*unsweetened*)	1 cup
Cream cheese (*non-dairy versions*)	2 tbsp
Diaya brand cheese (*tapioca base*)	1 oz
Feta cheese, Goat cheese	1 oz
Hummus	2 tbsp
Ketchup (*all natural, no sugar added*)	2 tbsp
Jam (*low sugar, no fake sweeteners*)	1 tbsp
Rice cheese, Soy cheese	1 oz or 1 slice
Vinaigrette dressing (*no dairy or wheat*)	2 tbsp
Any other food item that is less than 80 calories per serving, less than 5 g sugar, and gluten and dairy free	Varies

Cheat Foods

*Your cheat food can be anything you desire as long as it's gluten free and is under 300 calories. Remember that your Allowed Cheat Foods are measured in servings *per week* not serving per day. Here are some examples of cheat foods:

Food	Serving Size
Gluten-free pasta	2 oz
Beef tenderloin	3 oz
Dark chocolate	1 small bar
Wine, red or white	5 oz

Other foods that are allowed in unlimited quantities:

- Broth (beef, chicken, vegetable)
- Spices and seasonings (make sure they are gluten free)
- Unsweetened tea (hot or cold)
- Anything else that is calorie free (or under 20), gluten free, sugar free (no fake sugars or sweeteners except stevia), and not processed

The Importance of Tracking your Food

Whether you are following the sample meal plans or creating your meals, it is *essential* to keep track of what you eat in the nutrition logs I have provided. If you think writing down what you eat is pointless, or you just can't be bothered to do it, then consider this: studies have shown that, on average, people underestimate their daily caloric consumption by 30%-40%. No wonder we're all struggling to lose weight - we don't even know how much we're eating! There is a separate nutrition log for each phase that has empty rows for the exact number of foods allowed in each category. Once you have filled up each row, you're done with your food for the day. Make copies of your log sheets so that you have a fresh one for each day.

Remember, no one is looking at your log except you (unless you choose to share it with others), so be brutally honest. If you fall off the wagon and gorge yourself on muffins and bagels, write it down. Then take the next step of writing down how you felt afterwards, both physically and mentally. This is your chance to begin making the connection between what you eat and how you feel. Once you realize how much better you feel when you're off gluten, it will be that much easier to stick with the diet plan. Revel in feeling great!

Vegetables

Because I want your body to be nourished in the process of losing fat, **I'm requiring you to eat a minimum of five servings of vegetables per day**. We all have a tendency to eat protein and carbs for breakfast (eggs, bacon, bagels, cereal), more protein and carbs for lunch (sandwiches, wraps, tacos) and then arrive at dinner with exactly zero vegetables on board for the day. If you don't get in vegetables at breakfast, then you must start ticking off your required five a day by lunch or else you'll be forcing down cups of broccoli and spinach at dinner. All vegetables except for seven are considered "unlimited," which means you can eat as much as you want. The seven vegetables in the grey category have 5 grams or more of sugar per serving. **In Phase I you can have only one vegetable from the grey category per day, and by Phase III this increases to two.** Remember, on this diet you keep your total daily intake of sugar low, and I don't want you sabotaging your diet by eating too many high-sugar beets, carrots, potatoes, corn, and onions. **One final restriction on vegetables: no sauce, butter, or melted cheese on top.** Such toppings just take a healthy, low calorie food and turn it into a vehicle for unneeded calories and saturated fat.

Fruits

Unlike vegetables, I am putting restrictions on the total amount of fruit you eat each day. This may sound odd - fruit is supposed to be healthy for you, right? The answer is yes, but in moderation. Fruits provide a wonderful source of nutrients for our bodies, but they also provide fructose. Ah, here we are again talking about sugar. The three highest-sugar fruits per serving are apples, bananas, and watermelon. According to the 2011 Statistical Abstract of food consumption just released by the US government, the three most-eaten fruits in the United States are…..apples, bananas, and watermelon. We just can't get enough of sugar, no matter what form it takes! This is precisely why I've identified fruits that have more than 15 grams of sugar per serving and put those in the grey category.

In Phase I you can have only one fruit from the grey category per day, and by Phase III this increases to two. Technically you are allowed to have any fruit you choose outside the grey category until you reach the designated daily limit, but you should focus on the lowest-sugar fruits: blueberries, blackberries, raspberries, strawberries, and tangerines.

Protein

It may come as a surprise to you to find out that Americans actually eat *more* protein than they need - almost twice the amount recommended by the USDA. According to their recommendation, a healthy adult should consume 0.8 g of protein per kg of body weight. A person weighing 65kg (143 pounds) would therefore need 52 grams of protein per day. Most protein bars contain between 20-25 grams, a 4 ounce chicken breast contains 28 grams, and an egg has 7 grams. Voilá! You're already at the recommended daily amount.

For a 143-pound person, 52 grams of protein comes out to only 15% of a 1,400 calorie diet, which is slightly low in my experience. I'm going to have you consuming between 20%-25% of your calories from protein, the majority of which will come from very lean sources such as chicken and fish. Luckily there are some wonderfully lean red meat choices on the market today (i.e. 96% lean ground beef), but I'm putting all the high-fat cuts of meat in the grey category in order to ensure that you don't get too much saturated fat in your diet.

Protein rule #1: No fake or processed meats or fish. This means no imitation crab meat, processed sausages, or deli meats with additives. You will notice that I do have deli meat listed quite frequently as a snack in the sample meal plans, and I want you to purchase a brand that has no added nitrates, no fillers, and no added sugar. Look for brands that say things like "all-natural" and "low sodium" and "no added nitrates."

Protein rule #2: Beware of added sugar in protein foods. More often than not, those protein bars you are snacking on contain twice as many carbs as protein, and about 25-30 grams of added sugar. Yes, they may contain enticing-sounding things like amino acids and other minerals, but all the other additives cancel out the positive qualities. You may as well eat a Snickers bar and a multi-vitamin and call it even. The good news is that there are a few companies making natural, low sugar bars and drinks, but again be sure to check the carb and fat content. If you choose to have one of these items for a snack (I include *Mix 1* drinks as a snack in the meal plans) then you have to count it as an "other" food because all bars and drinks contain a mixture of carbs, proteins, and fats.

The other place to look for added sugar is in deli meats and bacon. Be sure to check the label for any of the sugar ingredients listed in Chapter 3 (essentially anything ending in"ose") and also beware of fake sugars and sweeteners. Just get the real stuff!

Dairy . . . or lack thereof

You will quickly notice that almost all dairy products are suspiciously absent from the "Allowed Proteins" list. Yes, this is intentional. I have two main reasons for excluding almost all forms of dairy from this diet. First, dairy products have a surprisingly high amount of sugar in them. After all, dairy contains lactose, an "ose" food, which we all know by now is just another sneaky way to describe sugar. Don't believe me? Consider a single serving (8 ounces) of fat free milk: it may be low in calories, but it contains 13 grams of sugar. In fact, all the low fat versions of your favorite dairy products have essentially swapped fat for sugar. And the full-fat versions contain a high amount of saturated fat, so they're no better.

The second reason I've excluded most dairy from this diet is that there is a strong connection between gluten allergies and dairy allergies. A large number of people who can't tolerate gluten also cannot tolerate dairy. My suspicion (which has been argued by other nutrition experts as well) is that the common denominator is sugar. We know from Chapter 3 that most gluten products contain a high amount of sugar, and since most dairy products do as well.....you see the connection. So what's a dairy-loving dieter to do? Simple: switch to non-dairy versions of the foods you know and love. There are some wonderful options on the market today such as rice cheese, soy cheese, almond cheese, even tapioca cheese. These same options are available for milk substitutions as well.

I have made exceptions for goat and feta cheese because they are significantly lower in sugar content and their allergen markers are lower as well. Additionally, I'm allowing Greek yogurt in all three phases of the diet. You've probably noticed that this type of yogurt is popping up next to your favorite Dannon flavors in the dairy section of the market, and the good news is that it's becoming more and more affordable as it gains popularity. Greek yogurt simply refers to the process of straining the yogurt twice. The second straining takes off all the unwanted sugar and carbohydrates and only leaves the good stuff: protein, probiotics, and calcium. In short, this stuff is a dieter's dreamboat.

Carbohydrates

This is not a low-carb diet, and in our current anti-carb climate I realize that statement may not be very popular. Carb is quite literally the four-letter word of the diet world, but this harmless source of energy has gotten a bad rap over the years. First of all, it's not carbs that make peo-

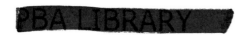

ple fat: it's carbohydrate-dense foods that are also loaded with refined sugar, saturated fat, and empty calories that make people fat (refer to Chapter 3 for a detailed explanation). You'll notice that there are no cupcakes, cookies, pastries, or desserts included in this diet. Instead, you'll be nourishing your body with complex carbohydrates that are high in fiber, free of refined sugar, and carefully spaced throughout the day to provide a steady, consistent source of energy.

Another reason to avoid low-carb diets is that they don't work on a long-term basis. If you're like millions of other Americans who have tried every diet gimmick on the market (myself included), you know that low-carb diets are extremely effective for initial weight loss, but extremely detrimental to sustained weight loss. In fact, most people who lose weight on a low-carb diet eventually gain that weight back *plus more*. To make matters worse, the weight that is gained back after a fad diet is almost always fat pounds, meaning that you end up with higher body fat after the diet than before. I have a feeling you may know what I'm talking about. You're probably reading this book because you've tried low-carb diets and yet here you are, still looking for a diet plan that you can actually sustain for longer than two weeks. Now that you know this isn't an unsustainable low-carb diet that will have you cursing my name and crying out for toast at 6 a.m., I'd like to show you how to include carbohydrates in your diet in a healthy way.

Carbohydrate rule #1: You must get a minimum of 48 grams of whole grains per day. This is in line with USDA's current recommendation, and I couldn't agree with it more. In fact, I would love to see you eat only whole grain sources, but I recognize this probably isn't realistic. However, be aware that eating whole grains is crucial to weight loss. I already explained the difference between whole grains and refined grains in Chapter 3, and now is your chance to see what an impact eating whole grains can have on your waistline. If you don't eat 48 grams of whole grains per day, then chances are you won't be getting enough fiber in your diet and your elimination (yes, I'm talking about poo) will not be efficient. To identify which foods contain whole grains, look for the Whole Grain stamp that has been issued by the Whole Grains Council.

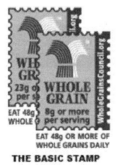

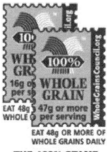

EAT 48g OR MORE OF WHOLE GRAINS DAILY

THE BASIC STAMP   **THE 100% STAMP**

Sometimes foods that are naturally whole grain will not carry the whole grain stamp. For example, the following gluten-free grains and grasses are naturally whole grain as well:

- Amaranth
- Brown rice
- Buckwheat
- Millet
- Oats
- Polenta
- Popcorn
- Quinoa
- Sorghum
- Teff
- Wild rice

From this list, the two options highest in protein are amaranth and quinoa. In fact, quinoa is a complete protein, which makes it a great choice for all you vegetarians out there who are following this plan. All of the options listed above are surprisingly easy to prepare, though many of them may be unfamiliar to you. When creating the meal plans, I assumed that most people reading this would be reluctant to try out new grains (we're all such creatures of habit, aren't we?), so I stuck to the ones that are most often found in the typical American diet: brown rice, oats, polenta, popcorn, quinoa, and wild rice. These food items are also easy to find in most markets, even if you live in a rural or remote area. If, however, you are feeling adventurous and want to take a culinary journey into the land of new grains, then by all means incorporate amaranth, buckwheat, millet, sorghum, and teff into your fat loss plan.

Carbohydrate rule #2: No more than 5 grams of sugar per serving in your grey category carbohydrates. This diet is pretty unique in that I allow you to eat such foods as bread, bagels, and waffles right from the start. However, I want you to be very careful when choosing your gluten-free bread products. Read your labels and make sure that the product you purchase (or make) does not contain more than 5 grams of sugar per serving. The last thing I want is for you to make the switch to a gluten-free diet and then inadvertently end up eating sugar-laden foods in the process. Furthermore, no fake sweeteners! The only sweeteners that are allowed are natural sugars, fruit sugars, and stevia.

Fats

The fats you will consume on this diet are derived predominantly from plant-based sources. What's a plant source? Anything that's not an animal. This means that instead of getting your fat from meat and dairy, you will get it from nuts, oils, olives, and avocados. For all of you carnivores out there getting nervous right now, don't worry - this diet is not vegetarian (unless you want it to be). It is, however, mindful of the fact that animal products are inherently higher in saturated fat than plant products.

Total allowed fat grams range between 35-45 grams per day. This is approximately two-thirds the amount recommended by the USDA, so please don't pay attention to the part of the food label that gives the "%Daily Value" because it doesn't apply to you. Also, don't be tempted to reduce the fat even more. Just as low-carb or no-carb diets aren't healthy or sustainable, neither are no-fat diets. Unsaturated fats are actually a critical component to our diet, and by excluding them we run the risk of sabotaging not only weight loss but also physical and mental well-being, not to mention satiety.

Other Foods

This is a catch-all category for foods that contain a combination of protein, fat, and/or carbs. For example, rice cheese slices are actually quite low in calories (only 40 per slice) but they contain an equal amount of carbs and protein, which puts them in the "other" category. In addition to foods that contain a mixture of macronutrients, you will also find snack foods, dressings, and spreads. **Though no single one of these items contains a large amount of calories, if you consume them indiscriminately throughout the day, those calories will add up.**

For example, think about how much ketchup you put on your sandwich. Realistically, it's probably somewhere in the 1/8 - 1/4 cup range, because that's what it takes to actually saturate the bread. Assuming you're eating the good ol Heinz brand, that 1/4 cup of ketchup contains a whopping 120 calories and 24 grams of added sugar. An extra 120 calories a day in your diet will add up to a weight gain of over 10 pounds per year - just from eating too much ketchup! Bottom line: don't be lax about tracking the foods in this category. They aren't freebies.

Cheat Foods

Finally, something indulgent! Cheat foods are exactly what they sound like - your opportunity to reward yourself for a week of hard work by eating one of your favorite items. What qualifies as a cheat food? Anything that's gluten free and yummy. Maybe you want a gluten-free brownie, maybe you're dying for some ice cream. The choice is yours, BUT.....**your cheat foods must adhere to the calorie restriction, which is 300 calories.** This may sound harsh, but the last thing you need is to ruin a week's worth of hard work with one super-rich, calorically-loaded meal that puts you right back to square one. Reward yourself, but keep your eyes on the finish line at the same time.

Water

We're all chronically dehydrated. The recommended minimum daily intake of water is 8 glasses, or 64 ounces. However, this amount is for sedentary individuals and people who are at a healthy body weight. If you are active or overweight, you'll need even more water. **A good formula is to divide your body weight in half and drink that many ounces a day of water.** For example, if you weigh 150 pounds, then you need to drink a minimum of 75 ounces of water each day. If you think that drinking water is a chore and you're not convinced of the value, look at some of the common symptoms of chronic dehydration:

- Excess weight and obesity
- Lack of energy
- Constipation
- Chronic headaches
- Allergies
- Eczema
- High blood pressure

You stopped at the "excess weight and obesity" one, didn't you? That's right, not drinking enough water can be a huge contributing factor to your inability to lose weight. One of the main reasons is that the body often confuses thirst for hunger, so you might be reaching for unhealthy snack foods when really your body is crying out for a simple glass of agua. So drink up! I've included 8 markers for your minimum 8 glasses of water at the top of each nutrition log. Be sure to mark each one off as you drink.

Bonnie's Gluten Free Fat Loss Story

I can honestly say that this program has been the most rewarding and positive lifestyle change I have ever made. I have been a compulsive eater my whole life, and have constantly struggled with my weight. Every single diet I've tried in the past left me feeling tired, hungry, depressed, or all three. And to complicate things even more, I don't cook. Seriously, my idea of cooking is heating things up in the microwave, so when I found out that Allison's plan had an entire set of meal plans for people like me I was thrilled!

Here are the hard numbers: **I lost 30 pounds in 3 months on the program, and I've kept it off.** The weight simply melted off - it's almost unbelievable how easy the program is to follow. I also kept track of my measurements with the Weekly Measurements page in the book, and I've lost a total of 16 inches. The other day I wore a tank top to the gym and I actually felt good in it! Here's another important aspect of the diet: I'm a very active runner, so I need energy for my long runs. Never once have I felt hungry on this plan or like I can't run because I don't have enough fuel. In fact, I've actually gotten faster and stronger in my workouts. I've also been religiously following the strength and flexibility plan in this book and I've been shocked at how fit I feel.

My friends, family, and co-workers are constantly stopping me and telling me how great I look, and they all want to know how I did it. I tell them it was the easiest, best-tasting diet plan in the world, and then I give them a copy of the book. Thank you Allison - you've changed my life!!

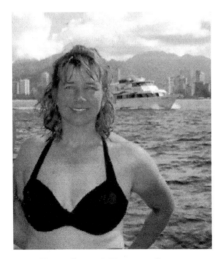

Bonnie at 165 pounds

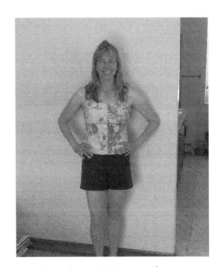

Bonnie at 135 pounds

Chapter 6

Sample Meal Plans

These meal plans will become an indispensable guide for most of you, especially when you're first starting the diet. **You can mix and match meals from different days and columns, but you must still track your food and adhere to the limits of the Daily Allowances for each Food Category.** For example, if you have the No Cooking breakfast on Day 2 (a bagel, which is a grey category carbohydrate) then you switch over to the Cooking column for dinner and eat the suggested Game Day Black Bean Burger, you'll need to skip the suggested two slices of gluten-free bread (also a grey carbohydrate) because in Phase I you're only allowed one grey carbohydrate per day. Did I already mention the importance of using the Nutrition Logs?

Though it's not required, I strongly suggest that you choose organic options whenever possible, and that you buy the whole-grain version of bread products and crackers. Remember that you're following this diet to make a positive difference in your health and well-being, and eating organic and whole-grain foods is just another step in that process.

Key for measurements and abbreviations used in the meal plans:

tsp= teaspoon
tbsp= tablespoon
oz= ounce

Phase I Meal Plans

All meals marked with an asterisk can be found in the recipe section

DAY 1

Meal	Cooking	No Cooking
Breakfast	1 serving Blueberry Almond Oatmeal*	6 oz non-fat Greek yogurt (*plain*), ¼ cup uncooked oatmeal (*less than 8g sugar*), ¼ cup sliced almonds, 1 tsp agave nectar *Combine all ingredients in one bowl and enjoy*
Morning Snack	2 tbsp hummus, 15 rice crackers or nut thins	Same
Lunch	Make your own salad: Mixed greens as base, ½ cup garbanzo beans, 1 tbsp chopped nuts, 6 oz chicken, any veggies you want (*not from grey category*), 2 tbsp low-fat vinaigrette dressing	Order this same salad from a restaurant or go to a salad bar
Afternoon Snack	1 hard-boiled egg, 1 serving of fruit	Same
Dinner	2 servings Crispy Potato Slices with Smoked Salmon and Cream Cheese*	*Amy's Organics* Frozen Enchilada Whole Meal (*non-dairy version*)

Daily Gluten-Free Tip: Sometimes gluten is added to salad dressings, so be sure to read the ingredient list. A few of my favorite gluten-free vinaigrettes are made by *Annie's* and *Newman's Own*.

DAY 2

Meal	Cooking	No Cooking
Breakfast	½ cup (raw measurement) slow cooking oatmeal, $^1/_8$ cup sliced nuts, ½ cup berries	1 gluten-free bagel (*under 300 calories*), 2 tbsp non-dairy cream cheese, ½ cup berries
Morning Snack	1 hard-boiled egg, 1 serving of fruit	Same
Lunch	Leftovers from Day 1 dinner: 1 serving Crispy Potato Slices with Salmon and Cream Cheese	Three fajita vegetable hard tacos from restaurant: *Only black beans, small amount of rice, corn salsa, fajita veggies, salsa*
Afternoon Snack	2 tbsp hummus, raw veggies of your choice (*not from grey category*)	Same
Dinner	1 serving Game Day Black Bean Burger* Allowed toppings: *1 slice non-dairy cheese, 2 slices whole grain gluten-free bread, mustard, pickles (no ketchup)* Side salad of mixed greens and veggies of your choice (*not from grey category*), 2 tbsp low-fat vinaigrette dressing	6 ounces salmon and steamed veggies from restaurant of your choice. (*keep track of your grey vegetables, no sauces*) ½ cup rice OR small baked potato (*no toppings on potato*)

Daily Gluten-Free Tip: Sometimes pre-made gluten-free bread products can be a little dry. Try popping them in the toaster or microwave for a few seconds to help create the softness and warmth of fresh-made bread.

DAY 3

Meal	Cooking	No Cooking
Breakfast	1 Banana Blueberry Muffin* 1 Breakfast Smoothie*	6 oz non-fat Greek yogurt (*plain*), 1 banana, ¼ cup uncooked oatmeal (*less than 8 g sugar*) *Combine all ingredients in one bowl and enjoy*
Morning Snack	2 tbsp hummus, 15 rice crackers or nut thins	Same
Lunch	Leftovers from Day 2 dinner: 1 serving Game Day Black Bean Burger (*same toppings allowed as last night*) Same side salad as last night OR steamed veggies	Grilled Chicken Breast salad from restaurant of your choice (*No cheese, no croutons, 2 tbsp low-fat vinaigrette dressing. Ask the server if the salad is gluten free.*)
Afternoon Snack	2 tbsp all-natural peanut or almond butter (*no sugar added*), 2 brown rice cakes	Same
Dinner	1 serving Spicy Red Pepper and Mushroom Enchiladas*	*Amy's Organics* Brown Rice and Veggie Bowl with Tofu

Daily Gluten-Free Tip: Two of the recipes in today's plan - the Banana Blueberry Muffins and the Spicy Red Pepper and Mushroom Enchiladas - freeze well. Now you have a ready-made dinner for those evenings when you get home late.

DAY 4

Meal	Cooking	No Cooking
Breakfast	1 Banana Blueberry Muffin* 1 egg, cooked to your liking	1 Breakfast Smoothie* (*in the recipe section- it's technically not cooking*)
Morning Snack	Mix 1 Protein drink (*or other protein drink with less than 5 g sugar per serving*)	Same
Lunch	Leftovers from Day 3 dinner: 1 serving Spicy Red Pepper and Mushroom Enchiladas	6 oz vegetable soup (*check ingredients for gluten*) 2 slices whole grain gluten-free bread
Afternoon Snack	3 brown rice cakes, 3 oz deli meat	Same
Dinner	1 serving Snow Pea, Pepper and Carrot Stir-Fry* 1 cup cooked brown rice	Sushi time! 1 roll of your choice (*no cream cheese, no tempura, tamari sauce in place of soy sauce*) Seaweed or side salad if desired (*confirm it is gluten free*)

Daily Gluten-Free Tip: Rice is a staple of most gluten-free diets, and investing in a rice cooker will make preparation and clean-up a breeze. Pick one up at Target for as little as $15.

DAY 5

Meal	Cooking	No Cooking
Breakfast	¼ cup (raw measurement) slow cooking oatmeal 1 serving of fruit, 1 egg (*cooked to your liking*)	1 packet instant oatmeal (*less than 8 g sugar*) made with hot water (*stevia for sweetener if desired*), 1 serving of fruit, 1 hard-boiled egg
Morning Snack	1 serving of fruit, 6 oz non-fat Greek yogurt (*plain*)	Same
Lunch	Leftovers from Day 4 dinner: 1 serving Snow Pea, Pepper, and Carrot Stir-Fry 1 cup cooked brown rice	1 cup Chicken and Green Chili soup from restaurant (*confirm it's gluten free*) Side salad with veggies of your choice (*no cheese, no croutons, 2 tbsp low-fat vinaigrette dressing*)
Afternoon Snack	15 rice crackers, 2 tbsp hummus	Same
Dinner	2 servings Tofu Spring Rolls* 1 cup cooked quinoa OR other gluten-free grain of your choice	Make or order two Turkey Sandwiches (*one is for lunch tomorrow*): 2 slices gluten-free bread, 4 oz turkey, any veggies, mustard, pickles (*no ketchup or mayo*) 2 servings of veggies (*only one from grey category*)

Daily Gluten-Free Tip: If you want to purchase hard boiled eggs for the No Cooking plan, you can find them at most grocery stores. However, making them at home is easy and saves you some money this way. Place 6-8 eggs in a large pot and fill it with enough water to cover the eggs. Turn the burner on medium-high and wait for the water to boil. Once boiling, set a timer for 10 minutes. After 10 minutes, drain off the water, then let the eggs cool in a bowl of cold water and ice.

DAY 6

Meal	Cooking	No Cooking
Breakfast	1 serving Cheesy Breakfast Tacos* 1 serving of fruit (*not from grey category*)	1 Breakfast smoothie*
Morning Snack	15 Veggie Chips (try Sweet Potato chips by *Terra*), 1 serving of fruit	Same
Lunch	Leftovers from Day 5 dinner: 2 servings Tofu Spring Rolls 1 cup cooked quinoa OR other gluten-free grain of your choice	The same gluten-free turkey sandwich you had for dinner yesterday.
Afternoon Snack	6 oz non-fat Greek yogurt (*plain*), ½ cup uncooked oatmeal	Same
Dinner	1 serving African Vegetable Stew with Raisins* 1 serving of carbohydrate (*it can be from grey category!*)	2 spring rolls or lettuce wraps from restaurant or grocery store (*Check ingredients for gluten, and be sure there is no added sugar. Buy 2 extras for lunch tomorrow*) 1 cup cooked brown rice OR other gluten-free grain of your choice

Daily Gluten-Free Tip: Today's Cooking breakfast is one of my all-time favorite recipes. I use Daiya brand cheese (cheddar style) because it melts perfectly. If your local store doesn't carry it, you can look up the nearest retailer at www.daiyafoods.com.

DAY 7

Meal	Cooking	No Cooking
Breakfast	1 serving Blueberry Almond Oatmeal*	1 gluten-free bagel (*less than 300 calories*), 2 oz smoked salmon, 2 tbsp non-dairy cream cheese
Morning Snack	6 oz non-fat Greek yogurt (*plain*), 1 serving of fruit (*not from grey category*)	Same
Lunch	Leftovers from Day 6 dinner: 1 serving African Vegetable Stew with Raisins 1 cup cooked quinoa OR other gluten-free grain of your choice	Leftovers: 2 spring rolls or lettuce wraps 1 cup cooked brown rice OR other gluten free grain of your choice
Afternoon Snack	1 hard-boiled egg, raw veggies of your choice (*not from grey category*)	Same
Dinner	Weekly cheat meal! (*see guidelines for cheat meal on p.54*)	Weekly cheat meal! (*see guidelines for cheat meal on p.54*)

Daily Gluten-Free Tip: Your cheat meal day is the perfect time to try out one of the yummy recipes from Phase II or III. This way you don't have to wait weeks before discovering the joy of gluten-free lasagna.

Shopping List for
Phase I Meal Plans Cooking

*Vegetables: salad greens, red peppers, mushrooms, snow peas, carrots, white potatoes, sweet potatoes, onions, tomatoes, spinach, frozen peas, vegetable broth

*Fruits: your choice, but focus on fruits from the non-grey category

*Proteins: non-fat, plain Greek yogurt (try *Fage* or *Oikos* brand), skinless chicken breast, deli meat (no nitrates, sugar, or fillers), eggs, extra firm tofu, smoked salmon

*Carbohydrates: slow cooking oatmeal, whole grain brown rice cakes, whole grain brown rice crackers, whole grain gluten-free sandwich bread and bagels, garbanzo beans, black beans, organic corn tortillas, brown rice or quinoa or any other gluten-free grain you prefer

*Non-dairy products: cream cheese, sliced cheese

*Fats: olive oil, sliced almonds, peanut butter or almond butter (no sugar added, all natural), peanut sauce (try *San-J*)

*Other foods: hummus (store-bought, or get ingredients for Allison's Secret Hummus), low-fat vinaigrette salad dressing, enchilada sauce (no sugar added, gluten free), rice papers, small container of raisins

*Spices and herbs: cinnamon, red pepper, salt and pepper, cilantro

Shopping List for
Phase I Meal Plans, No Cooking

*Vegetables: raw veggies of your choice (you can get pre-cut veggies, or cut them up yourself), mixed greens, vegetable soup

*Fruits: your choice, but focus on fruits from the non-grey category

*Proteins: non-fat, plain Greek yogurt (try *Fage* or *Oikos* brand), hard boiled eggs, deli meat (no sugar added, nitrate free, no fillers), smoked salmon, protein powder (less than 3 g sugar per serving, no artificial ingredients or sweeteners)

*Carbohydrates: instant oatmeal (less than 8 g sugar per serving), whole grain rice crackers, whole grain rice cakes, whole grain gluten-free sandwich bread and bagels

*Fats: nuts of your choice, almond or peanut butter (no sugar added, all natural)

*Other foods: agave nectar, hummus, non-dairy cream cheese, unsweetened almond milk, low fat vinaigrette salad dressing, Larabar or KIND bar or Mix 1 drinks

Amy's Organics* **Frozen meals: Whole Meal Enchilada, Tamale Verde (non dairy), Brown Rice and Veggie Bowl with Tofu, any other varieties that are gluten and dairy free. Your frozen meals can be a different brand than *Amy's Organics*, but they need to be all-natural with no preservatives or sugar added.

Phase I Nutrition Log

(Make copies of this page and fill one out each day)

Date:_____   Day on GF Fat Loss Plan: _____

Glasses of water: 1 2 3 4 5 6 7 8

(1 glass=8 ounces)

Vegetable	Serving size	Notes

Fruit	Serving size	Notes

Protein	Serving size	Notes

Carbohydrate*	Serving size	Notes

Fat	Serving Size	Notes

Other food	Serving Size	Notes

Cheat food	Serving size	Notes

*Make sure at least 2 of your carbohydrate choices are whole grain.

Phase II Meal Plans

All meals marked with an asterisk can be found in the recipe section

DAY 1

Meal	Cooking	No Cooking
Breakfast	1 serving Blueberry Almond Oatmeal*	1 packet instant oatmeal (*less than 8 g sugar*) made with hot water (*stevia for sweetener if desired*), 1 serving of fruit, 2 tbsp almonds
Morning Snack	3 oz deli meat, 1 oz almond cheese	Same
Lunch	4 oz grilled chicken breast, 1 serving of vegetables (*no grey category*), 1 small baked potato (*no toppings except salsa*)	Order this same meal from a restaurant. You can substitute 1 cup cooked brown rice for the potato if necessary.
Afternoon Snack	2 brown rice cakes, 2 tbsp baba ghanoush spread or hummus	Same
Dinner	1 serving Baked Butternut Squash, Apples and Walnuts* 1 cup cooked wild rice OR other gluten-free grain of your choice (*I love to spoon the Squash recipe on top of wild rice- yum!*)	Order 4 spinach and mushroom enchiladas from a restaurant (*no cheese, no sour cream, tortillas must be corn, add 4 oz goat cheese if desired*). Save 2 enchiladas for lunch tomorrow.

Daily Gluten-Free Tip: Baba ghanoush is a spread typically seen in Middle Eastern cuisine, but you can find it at most grocery stores. It's very similar to hummus, except that hummus is made with pureed chick peas and baba ghanoush is made with pureed eggplant. What a great way to sneak in an extra serving of veggies!

DAY 2

Meal	Cooking	No Cooking
Breakfast	Breakfast sandwich: 1 gluten-free bagel *(less than 300 calories)* 2 scrambled egg whites, 1 oz or 1 slice non-dairy cheese *(I use almond cheese)*	1 gluten-free bagel *(less than 300 calories)*, 2 tbsp low sugar jam, 2 tbsp non-dairy cream cheese
Morning Snack	2 tbsp hummus, raw veggies of your choice *(not from grey category)*	Same
Lunch	Leftovers from Day 1 dinner: 1 serving Baked Butternut Squash, Apples, and Walnuts 1 cup cooked wild rice OR other gluten-free grain of your choice	Leftovers from Day 1 dinner: 2 spinach and mushroom enchiladas
Afternoon Snack	1 hard-boiled egg, 1 serving of fruit *(not from grey category)*	Same
Dinner	1 serving Gluten-free Meatballs* 1 serving Roasted Brussels Sprouts with Dates*	From restaurant or frozen section of grocery store: 3 oz turkey burger, 2 slices gluten-free bread, any veggies, mustard, pickles *(no ketchup or mayo)* Side salad with veggies of your choice *(no cheese, no croutons, 2 tbsp low-fat vinaigrette dressing)*

Daily Gluten-Free Tip: If you have committed to the Cooking column of the meal plans, then you'll be spending time chopping up ingredients for recipes. Nothing takes the joy out of cooking like wrestling with a dull knife blade, so be sure to keep your knives sharpened. Don't want to deal with the hassle? Try a Yoshi blade, which will cut through anything and never gets dull.

DAY 3

Meal	Cooking	No Cooking
Breakfast	1 Blueberry Banana Muffin* 2 scrambled egg whites	1 gluten-free frozen waffle, 2 tsp agave nectar, 1 serving of fruit
Morning Snack	15 rice crackers, 2 oz almond cheese	Same
Lunch	Leftovers from Day 2 dinner: 1 serving Gluten-free Meatballs 1 serving Roasted Brussels Sprouts with Dates	From restaurant: 4 oz plain hamburger (*no bun*) or chicken breast, 1 small baked potato (*no toppings except salsa*) Side salad or steamed veggies (*same side salad rules you've seen before*)
Afternoon Snack	1 serving sweet potato chips (try *Terra Chips* brand)	Same
Dinner	1 serving Baked Halibut with Strawberry Cilantro Salsa* ½ cup cooked brown or wild rice	From restaurant or prepared foods section of grocer: 6 oz grilled or baked fish, unlimited veggies (*no butter or sauce on either*) 1 cup cooked brown or wild rice

Daily Gluten-Free Tip: When ordering a salad, ask if the salad dressing is gluten free and make sure the protein (chicken, shrimp, etc.) hasn't been dusted with flour.

DAY 4

Meal	Cooking	No Cooking
Breakfast	2 gluten-free frozen waffles, 2 tsp agave nectar	1 packet instant oatmeal (*less than 8 g sugar*) made with hot water (*stevia for sweetener if desired*), 1 serving of fruit, 2 tbsp almonds
Morning Snack	3 oz deli meat, raw veggies of your choice (*not from grey category*)	Same
Lunch	Leftovers from Day 3 dinner: 1 serving Baked Halibut with Strawberry Cilantro Salsa ½ cup cooked brown or wild rice	Any Indian dish that is gluten-free and dairy-free (*goat or feta cheese are allowed*). Measure out a circle that is 6" in diameter and only eat that much. Take the rest home for leftovers.
Afternoon Snack	1 serving of fruit, 1 tbsp nut butter	Same
Dinner	1 serving Roasted Eggplant Roll-ups* 2 oz (*dry measurements*) gluten-free pasta (*try Tinkyada brand, cook pasta according to package directions*) ½ cup pasta sauce (*no sugar added*)	Leftovers from lunch!

Daily Gluten-Free Tip: For your morning snack, trying putting sugar snap peas on a slice of deli ham or turkey and rolling it up - it makes a nice crunch!

DAY 5

Meal	Cooking	No Cooking
Breakfast	1 Breakfast Smoothie* 1 Blueberry Banana Muffin*	Same, but substitute 2 slices gluten-free toast if you don't want to make the muffins
Morning Snack	1 hard-boiled egg, 1 serving of fruit (*not from grey category*)	Same
Lunch	Leftovers from Day 4 dinner: 1 serving Roasted Eggplant Roll-ups 2 oz (*dry measurement*) gluten-free pasta ½ cup pasta sauce (*no sugar added*)	6 oz gluten-free vegetable soup (*add 3 oz protein if desired*) 2 warm corn tortillas
Afternoon Snack	2 tbsp hummus, raw veggies of your choice (*not from grey category*)	Same
Dinner	1 serving Apple, Chicken and Goat Cheese Salad*	Same (*the recipe is really just assembly*) OR order a grilled chicken and goat cheese salad from a restaurant (*as always, 2 tbsp low-fat vinaigrette dressing, and no croutons*)

Daily Gluten-Free Tip: If your friends and colleagues ask why you're eating gluten free, tell them how great you feel on the Gluten Free Fat Loss Plan, and challenge them to join you. A little friendly competition can be helpful.

DAY 6

Meal	Cooking	No Cooking
Breakfast	1 serving Traditional Farmer's Breakfast*	Go out for breakfast! Order 2 eggs, a side of fruit, and a half order of hash browns (*make sure they're gluten free*).
Morning Snack	2 brown rice cakes, 2 oz almond cheese	Same
Lunch	Leftovers from Day 5 dinner: 1 serving Apple, Chicken and Goat Cheese Salad	Salad: Have leftovers from last night OR try a mixed salad with shrimp, salmon or grilled chicken, and any veggies you want (*no cheese except feta or goat, no croutons, 2 tbsp low-fat vinaigrette dressing*)
Afternoon Snack	3 oz deli meat, 1 serving of fruit (*not from grey category*)	Same
Dinner	1 serving Crispy Polenta Cakes with Sundried Tomatoes and Kale*	Try to keep today's dinner vegetarian. Go for a small baked potato or sweet potato with ½ cup black beans, ½ cup cooked brown rice, ¼ cup salsa, and cilantro. Throw on 2 oz non-dairy, feta, or goat cheese if desired.

Daily Gluten-Free Tip: Today's Cooking dinner may involve some ingredients that are a little out of your comfort zone, but I guarantee you'll become a fan of kale after you taste this recipe. My friends frequently request this recipe when they come over for dinner.

DAY 7

Meal	Cooking	No Cooking
Breakfast	1 serving Blueberry Almond Oatmeal*	1 packet instant oatmeal (*less than 8 g sugar*) made with hot water (*stevia for sweetener if desired*), 1 serving of fruit, 2 tbsp almonds
Morning Snack	2 tbsp hummus, raw veggies of your choice (*not from grey category*)	Same
Lunch	Leftovers from Day 6 dinner: 1 serving Crispy Polenta Cakes with Sundried Tomatoes and Kale	Make or order a gluten-free Turkey Sandwich: 4 oz turkey, 2 slices gluten-free bread, any veggies, mustard, pickles (*no ketchup or mayo*) Side salad (*no cheese except goat or feta, no croutons, 2 tbsp low-fat vinaigrette dressing*)
Afternoon Snack	3 oz deli meat, 15 rice crackers	Same
Dinner	Cheat Meal! Try the Almond Crust Pizza with Mushrooms, Roma tomatoes, and Fresh Basil* You can even have a glass of red wine.	Cheat Meal! Find one of the many gluten-free pizza offerings in the frozen foods section, or at a local pizzeria. Remember, still no cheese except goat or feta. Top it off with a glass of red wine.

Daily Gluten-Free Tip: The cheat meal day is a great time to go out with friends. They'll be shocked (and jealous) when they see you drinking a glass of wine and eating delicious food while on a "diet"!

Shopping List for
Phase II Meal Plans, Cooking

*Vegetables: butternut squash, asparagus, mushrooms, white potato, Brussels sprouts, egg-plant, kale, dates, sundried tomatoes, onion, garlic, carrots, frozen hashbrowns (check for gluten)

*Fruits: blueberries, bananas, Granny Smith apples, strawberries, any other fruits you want to snack on

*Proteins: non-fat, plain Greek yogurt (try *Fage* or *Oikos* brand), skinless chicken breast, halibut, ground beef (96% lean), ground pork (leanest option available), bacon, deli meat (no added sugar, no nitrates, no fillers), eggs, almond cheese

*Carbohydrates: oats or oatmeal (try *Bob's Red Mill*), whole grain gluten-free bagels and bread, gluten-free bread crumbs (can buy these or crumble up some stale gluten-free bread), whole grain gluten-free pasta (try *Tinkyada*), polenta (get the tube kind), brown rice or quinoa or millet

*Fats: nut butter (all natural, no sugar added)

*Other: goat or feta cheese, rice or soy cheese slices, balsamic vinegar, ketchup (no sugar added), low-fat vinaigrette salad dressing, molasses, Terra chips (if these aren't available then get baked tortilla chips)

*Spices: fresh basil, fresh cilantro, sea salt, baking soda, cinnamon, vanilla, parsley

Shopping List for
Phase II Meal Plans, No Cooking

*Vegetables: raw veggies of your choice (you can get pre-cut veggies, or cut them up yourself)

*Fruits: your choice, but focus on non-grey category fruits

*Proteins: non-fat, plain Greek yogurt (try *Fage* or *Oikos* brand), hard boiled eggs, smoked salmon, almond cheese, protein powder, deli meat (no sugar added, no nitrates, no fillers)

*Carbohydrates: gluten-free instant oatmeal (less than 8 grams sugar per serving), whole grain rice crackers, whole grain rice cakes, whole grain gluten-free bagels and sandwich bread

*Fats: sliced almonds, nut butter (no sugar added, all natural)

*Other: agave nectar, hummus, non-dairy cream cheese spread, unsweetened almond milk, Larabar or KIND bar, low-fat vinaigrette dressing, feta or goat cheese

**Amy's Organics* Frozen Meals: technically there are no prescribed frozen meals in Phase II. However, it's a good idea to keep a few of these quick meals on hand just in case your original meal plans get derailed.

Phase II Nutrition Log

(Make copies of this page and fill one out each day)

Date:_____   Day on GF Fat Loss Plan: _____

Glasses of water: 1 2 3 4 5 6 7 8

(1 glass=8 ounce)

Vegetable	Serving size	Notes

Fruit	Serving size	Notes

Protein	Serving size	Notes

Carbohydrate*	Serving size	Notes

Fat	Serving Size	Notes

Other food	Serving Size	Notes

Cheat food	Serving size	Notes

*Make sure at least 2 of your carbohydrates choices are whole grain.

Phase III Meal Plans

All meals marked with an asterisk can be found in the recipe section

DAY 1

Meal	Cooking	No Cooking
Breakfast	1 serving Blueberry Almond Oatmeal*	1 packet instant oatmeal (*less than 8 g sugar*) made with hot water (*stevia for sweetener if desired*), 1 serving of fruit, ¼ cup sliced almonds
Morning Snack	1 hard-boiled egg, raw veggies of your choice (*only 1 from grey category*)	Same
Lunch	Make a grilled chicken or shrimp salad: Unlimited greens, veggies of your choice (*only 1 from grey category*), 3 oz protein (*still no croutons, no cheese except goat or feta, 2 tbsp low-fat vinaigrette dressing*) 1 cup cooked brown rice OR other gluten-free grain of your choice	Order this same meal from a restaurant
Afternoon Snack	15 brown rice crackers, 2 tbsp hummus	Same
Dinner	1 serving Gluten-free Meatballs* 2 oz (*dry measurement*) gluten-free pasta (*try Tinkyada brand, cook pasta according to package directions*) ½ cup pasta sauce (*no sugar added*)	*Amy's Organics* frozen Matar Paneer meal

Daily Gluten-Free Tip: If you just made the switch to Phase III, you'll notice that today's meal plan contains some familiar meals, but some of the serving sizes have been changed. This is intentional. Don't be afraid to enjoy your much deserved additional calories. You've earned it!

DAY 2

Meal	Cooking	No Cooking
Breakfast	1 serving Traditional Farmer's Breakfast*	*Amy's Organics* Cream of Rice Bowl, stir ½ scoop vanilla protein powder into rice bowl after it's heated
Morning Snack	1 Get Yer Veggies Smoothie* 2 brown rice cakes	8 oz V8 100% vegetable juice 2 brown rice cakes
Lunch	Leftovers from Day 1 dinner: 1 serving Gluten-free Meatballs Large side salad (you know how to make this by now- same parameters as Phase II)	From Chipotle-type restaurant: Chicken burrito bowl *Black beans, rice, chicken, lettuce, salsa, guacamole. No cheese or sour cream, no chips. Eat half of the bowl, take other half home for lunch tomorrow*
Afternoon Snack	6 oz non-fat Greek yogurt (*plain*), ½ cup dry oatmeal	6 oz non-fat Greek yogurt (*plain*), ¼ cup sliced nuts
Dinner	1 serving Almond Chicken Cutlets with Mango* 1 medium baked potato (*no toppings except salsa, goat cheese, or feta cheese*)	From restaurant or frozen food section: 4 oz turkey burger (*no bun, no cheese, veggie toppings are allowed*) Side salad or steamed veggies 1 small serving sweet potato fries or regular fries

Daily Gluten-Free Tip: Now that you're in the maintenance phase, it can be tempting to loosen up the belt on your gluten-free lifestyle. Stay focused and remember: Loosening up the belt on anything in your life (especially your pants) is something you never want to do again!

DAY 3

Meal	Cooking	No Cooking
Breakfast	1 Pre-Workout Shake*	Same, or Mix 1 Protein drink (*any flavor*)
Morning Snack	3 oz sliced turkey, 2 brown rice cakes, 2 tbsp hummus	Same
Lunch	Leftovers from Day 2 dinner: 1 serving Almond Chicken Cutlets with Mango 1 medium baked potato (*no toppings except salsa, goat cheese, or feta cheese*)	Leftovers from yesterday's lunch OR 1 can (10 oz) gluten-free chili, 1 slice gluten-free bread
Afternoon Snack	1 hard-boiled egg, raw veggies of your choice (*only 1 from grey category*)	Same
Dinner	4 oz broiled salmon, 1 cup cooked brown or wild rice, steamed green beans (*as much as you want*)	Sushi: 1 roll of your choice (*no cream cheese or tempura, tamari instead of soy sauce,*) ½ cup edamame, side seaweed salad (*ask if the dressing is gluten-free*)

Daily Gluten-Free Tip: If you haven't already done so, today is a great day to try waking up early and eating your breakfast, then completing your workout before you head into the office.

DAY 4

Meal	Cooking	No Cooking
Breakfast	1 serving Spinach and Mushroom Scramble with Gluten-free Toast and Jam*	Hit your local diner for breakfast! Egg white omelet *(any veggies you want, feta or goat cheese)*, side order of fruit, ½ serving hashbrowns *(ask if they're gluten-free, and go easy on the ketchup)*
Morning Snack	1 tbsp nut butter, 1 serving of fruit *(try putting almond butter on a banana)*	Same
Lunch	Leftovers from Day 3 dinner: 4 oz broiled salmon, 1 cup cooked brown or wild rice, steamed green beans *(as much as you want)*	Order this same meal from restaurant
Afternoon Snack	1 serving baked tortilla chips, ¼ cup black bean salsa	Same
Dinner	1 serving Broccoli Quinoa* 4 oz grilled pork chop *(make an extra one for lunch tomorrow)*	Assemble a wrap: 1 large brown rice tortilla, 4 oz sliced turkey, any veggies you want, 2 tbsp hummus, mustard *(make an extra wrap for lunch tomorrow)*

Daily Gluten-Free Tip: It's time for me to break one of my own rules. Now that you're in Phase III, you can add ½ tbsp of dairy-free butter to your steamed vegetables. I like Earth Balance, which offers different flavor varieties. Enjoy!

DAY 5

Meal	Cooking	No Cooking
Breakfast	1 serving gluten-free hot cereal (*try Bob's Red Mill*), 1 egg, 1 serving of fruit	1 gluten-free bagel (*less than 300 calories per bagel*), 2 tbsp dairy-free cream cheese, sliced strawberries on top
Morning Snack	Mix 1 protein drink (*any flavor*)	Same
Lunch	Leftovers from Day 4 dinner: 1 serving Broccoli Quinoa 4 oz pork chop	Leftovers from Day 4 dinner: Turkey wrap, 1 serving of fruit
Afternoon Snack	2 brown rice cakes, 2 oz sliced turkey, 1 oz almond cheese	Same
Dinner	1 serving Gluten-free Lasagna* Large side salad, any veggies you want (*no croutons, no cheese except goat or feta, 2 tbsp low-fat vinaigrette dressing*)	1 serving frozen gluten-free lasagna (try *Amy's Organics* or *Cedarlane*) Large side salad, any veggies you want (*no croutons, no cheese except goat or feta, 2 tbsp low-fat vinaigrette dressing*)

Daily Gluten-Free Tip: Lasagna is one of the signature gluten dishes that people always tell me they can't live without. Now you don't have to - try taking this dish to a party or social gathering, but don't tell anyone it's gluten-free until after they have eaten it. Get ready for some looks of disbelief!

DAY 6

Meal	Cooking	No Cooking
Breakfast	Banana and Almond Butter Toast: 2 slices gluten-free toast (*not too thick*), 1 tbsp almond butter, ½ sliced banana on top	2 frozen gluten-free waffles (*try Van's buckwheat berry variety*), 2 tsp agave nectar
Morning Snack	15 brown rice crackers, 2 tbsp hummus, raw veggies of your choice	Same
Lunch	Leftovers from Day 5 dinner: 1 serving Gluten-free Lasagna Large side salad, any veggies you want (*no croutons, no cheese except goat or feta, 2 tbsp low-fat vinaigrette dressing*)	Soup and rice: 1 ½ cups bean and vegetable soup, 1 cup cooked brown rice
Afternoon Snack	6 oz non-fat Greek yogurt (*plain*), ½ cup raw oatmeal, ½ cup sliced strawberries	Same
Dinner	1 serving Grilled Turkey Sandwich* (*make an extra one for tomorrow*) 2 servings steamed veggies (*melt 1 oz almond cheese on top of veggies - rule violator! You've earned it!*)	Large salad: 4 oz chicken or fish, unlimited veggies, 2 oz goat or feta cheese, 2 tbsp vinaigrette dressing

Daily Gluten-Free Tip: You've made it this far, so it's clear that you are committed to your gluten-free lifestyle. Make the investment in a bread-making machine so that you can enjoy the soft, elastic texture of homemade gluten-free bread.

DAY 7

Meal	Cooking	No Cooking
Breakfast	2 small gluten-free pancakes from mix (*try The Gluten Free Pantry*) OR 2 gluten-free frozen waffles, 2 tsp agave nectar, 1 egg	Larabar (*any flavor with less than 18 g sugar*) OR KIND bar, 1 hard-boiled egg
Morning Snack	2 tbsp baba ghanoush or hummus, raw veggies of your choice	Same
Lunch	Leftovers from Day 6 dinner: 1 serving Grilled Turkey Sandwich Unlimited steamed veggies of your choice	Order a chicken sandwich from any deli or restaurant, but bring two slices of gluten-free bread (*no cheese except goat or feta, no mayo, any veggies you want*) Side salad (*remember your salad rules!*) OR steamed veggies
Afternoon Snack	1 serving sweet potato chips (try *Terra* brand)	Same
Dinner	Cheat meal!	Cheat meal!

Daily Gluten-Free Tip: Congrats - you are officially living a life of gluten free-dom! As you maintain your fat loss, know that falling off the gluten-free wagon once in a while doesn't mean you should throw in the towel for good. If you're feeling unsteady about your food choices, return to Phase II for a few days to get yourself back on track, and don't forget to fill out your Nutrition Logs.

Shopping List for
Phase III Meal Plans, Cooking

*Vegetables: onion, carrots, spinach, mushrooms, white potato, green beans, garlic, lots of raw veggies for snacks

*Fruits: mango, blueberries, strawberries, any other fruit you like

*Proteins: Non-fat, plain Greek yogurt (try *Fage* or *Oikos*),skinless chicken breast, ground pork (leanest variety available), ground beef (96% lean), bacon, salmon, eggs, extra firm tofu, protein powder

*Carbohydrates: oats or oatmeal (try *Bob's Red Mill*), whole grain gluten-free bagels and bread, whole grain gluten-free brown rice crackers and cakes, whole grain gluten-free pasta (one box lasagna noodles, one box any other noodle of your choice - try *Tinkyada* brand), frozen hashbrowns (check for gluten ingredients) brown rice (can sub millet or quinoa) , brown rice flour

*Fats: olive oil, nut butter (all natural, no sugar added), sliced nuts

*Other: low-fat vinaigrette salad dressing, hummus and/or baba ghanoush spread, large jar of pasta sauce (no sugar added), black bean salsa, baked chips or *Terra* chips, molasses, low fat coconut milk, non-dairy mozzarella cheese shreds (try *Galaxy* or *Daiya* brand), low sugar jam (try *Smuckers* or *Trader Joe's*), goat or feta cheese

*Spices: cinnamon, parsley, sea salt, pepper, apple cider vinegar, nutritional yeast

Shopping List for
Phase III Meal Plans, No Cooking

*Vegetables: lots of raw veggies for snacks, pre-made salad mix, V8 100% vegetable juice

*Fruits: blueberries, strawberries, bananas, and any other fruit you like

*Proteins: non-fat, plain Greek yogurt (try *Fage* or *Oikos*), hard boiled eggs, sliced deli meat (organic, no added nitrates or sugar), protein powder, Mix 1 protein drink (your choice of flavor)

*Carbohydrates: Gluten-free instant oatmeal (must be less than 8 g sugar per serving), whole grain brown rice crackers and cakes, whole grain gluten-free bagels, sandwich bread, and waffles

*Fats: sliced nuts, nut butter

*Other: low-fat vinaigrette salad dressing, hummus and/or baba ghanoush spread, dairy-free options (cream cheese, slices of rice, almond, or soy cheese for snacks and sandwiches), black bean salsa, baked chips or *Terra* chips, Larabar or KIND bar (must be less than 18 g sugar), low sugar jam (try *Smuckers* or *Trader Joe's*), goat or feta cheese

*Pre-made soup: chili and some variety of Tuscan bean soup (check for gluten ingredients)

Amy's Organics frozen meals: Hot Cereal Steel Cut Oats, Gluten-free Vegetable Lasagna, Matar Paneer

Phase III Nutrition Log

(Make copies of this page and fill one out each day)

Date:_____   **Day on GF Fat Loss Plan:** _____

Glasses of water: 1 2 3 4 5 6 7 8(1 glass=8 ounces)

Vegetable	Serving size	Notes

Fruit	Serving size	Notes

Protein	Serving size	Notes

Carbohydrate*	Serving size	Notes

Fat	Serving Size	Notes

Other food	Serving Size	Notes

Cheat food	Serving size	Notes

*Make sure at least 3 of your carbohydrate choices are whole grain.

Chapter 7

The Workout Program

You may have purchased this book for the sole purpose of losing weight by changing what you eat, but diet is only one part of a larger picture of health and wellness. Think of eating well as the base coat you apply to the canvas; it establishes what you're trying to create and helps to illuminate the overall vision. However, no picture is complete until you apply the top coat, the final adhesive that helps "set" the picture and ensures that it doesn't change or fade over time. This top coat is fitness. Regular exercise not only assists with continued weight loss, it helps keep your muscles, joints, lungs, and heart strong, and it gives you added energy. Our bodies were built to move, so get off the couch and start sweating!

As with the diet plan, my philosophy towards exercise is that it must be realistic or it won't work. That's why I've created three different levels from which to choose. **Your workout phase and your diet phase don't have to match:** You can be in Workout Phase I and Diet Phase II at the same time. After all, you may be one of those people who already works out regularly, yet still isn't seeing your body change. In this case, you would start with Workout Phase III and Diet Phase I. If you feel that you fall somewhere between workout phases, start with the lower phase first and then you can quickly switch to the next phase if you find it's too easy.

Phase I Workout:
- For people who have never been on a regular workout program, or who have not exercised regularly in the past six months
- For people who have limited time to devote to exercise

Phase II Workout:
- For people who have been on Phase I for at least three weeks
- For people who already exercise at least three days a week for 30 minutes or more
- For people who have exercised regularly within the last six months

Phase III Workout:
- For people who have been on Phase II for at least three weeks
- For people who already exercise at least four days a week for 45 minutes or more

The Three Components of the Workout Plan:
Cardio, Flexibility, and Core Strength

All of the **Cardio Workouts** will have a duration (amount of time) as well as Rate of Perceived Exertion (RPE) assigned to them. What exactly is a **Cardio Workout**? It's anything that involves constant movement and gets your heart rate up. Maintaining an elevated heart rate is the true foundation of gaining fitness and losing pounds. Unless you're a professional body-builder who lifts weight three hours a day, it is very difficult to decrease your body fat and drop pounds without doing cardio, and this is because cardio workouts burn a high amount of calories in a short amount of time, and we all know that in order to lose weight you have to burn more calories than you consume. Here are some examples of cardio workouts:

- Running
- Cycling
- Swimming
- Hiking
- Brisk walking
- Dancing
- Elliptical or other gym machines (Stair master, stationary bike, etc)
- Rowing
- Ice skating, Roller skating, Roller blading
- Tennis
- Rock climbing
- Aerobics, Kickboxing, or other group fitness classes
- Soccer, Volleyball, Basketball, or any other team sport
- Anything else you enjoy doing that involves constant movement!

The most important consideration when choosing a cardio activity is to pick something you enjoy. Exercise shouldn't be something you dread - it should be an activity that makes you smile. There will, of course, be days when your workout feels like a chore, but you will inevitably be glad you did it once you're done. I also encourage you to try something new with your cardio workouts and to switch up your activity on a regular basis. This will not only keep you from getting bored, it will also challenge your body in different ways and utilize a variety of muscle groups, which will decrease your chances of developing a repetitive use injury.

Each cardio workout also has a **Rate of Perceived Exertion** level assigned to it. This will take the guess work out of how hard you should be working, and it will also keep you honest about the intensity of your workout. **Rate of Perceived Exertion, or RPE,** is a subjective means of gauging how hard you're working. It is measured on a scale of 1-10.

RPE Number	Your level of effort	Example/Explanation
1	Very easy	Watching TV
2	Easy	Gentle walking
3	Moderate	Brisk walking
4	Moderate/Heavy	Easy jog
5	Slightly uncomfortable	Medium jog
6	Heavy effort	Getting difficult to talk
7	Very heavy effort	Fast jog/Sweating profusely
8	Difficult	Short sprint/Can't talk at all
9	Very difficult	Sprinting uphill/Muscles and lungs are burning
10	Extremely difficult/Impossible	Unable to go on/Lightheadedness/Vomiting

If you are using the RPE scale for the first time, it may seem confusing. You may wonder if you are supposed to gauge your level of exertion on how hard you are breathing, or how much your muscles and joints hurt, or how fatigued you feel overall - the answer is yes, yes, and yes. All three areas must be taken into consideration when gauging your level of effort. Your muscle fatigue might feel like a 7 while your breathing feels like a 3, or vice versa. With time and conditioning these numbers will start to move closer together, but when you are first embarking on your new workout program I advise you to honor the higher number (7 in this example) and take breaks when necessary in order to give your muscles and lungs a chance to recover. In Phase I you will never work harder than a 6 on the RPE scale because I want you to really focus on regulating your breathing and giving your muscles the necessary opportunity to tone up and gain strength. In Phase II you will begin to push into what is called the "anaerobic zone" by completing some interval training workouts that take you to a 7-8 on the RPE scale. In Phase III you will work in the anaerobic zone more frequently, but I won't ask you to go higher than an 8 unless you truly feel like your body and mind are ready.

Flexibility is also a critical part of your fitness routine. You may be curious (and disappointed) about my choice of focusing on flexibility. After all, it doesn't really get your heart rate up or burn calories, plus it can be insufferably boring. However, in my 10 plus years of working with clients of all ages and athletic abilities, I have found that all of them have one thing in common: poor posture. What most people don't realize is that poor posture is largely the result of certain muscle groups being too tight while others are too loose, which causes muscles to get "stuck" and inhibits them from firing properly and keeping your skeleton (i.e. your spine, your hips, your knees, etc) in its optimum position.

Picture someone who has a pronounced shoulder slouch. In the exercise physiology world this is called *Upper Cross Syndrome,* and it's characterized by forward shoulders, a concave chest, and a forward head carriage (chin being pushed abnormally far in front of the shoulders).

When *Upper Cross Syndrome* is present, it means that the following muscles are tight:

- Pectoralis major and minor
- Levator scapulae
- Teres major
- Upper trapezius
- Anterior deltoid
- Subscapularis
- Latissimus dorsi
- Sternocleidomastoid
- Rectus capitus
- Scalenes

And the following muscles are loose and overstretched:

- Rhomboids
- Lower trapezius
- Serratus anterior
- Posterior deltoid
- Teres minor
- Infraspinatus
- Longus coli/capitus

Since all of those muscle names are very hard to pronounce and spell, not to mention locate on the body, here is a simple summary: all of the tight muscles are on the *front side* of the body (there are just a few that are on the back, but they still pull you forward) and all of the loose muscles are on the *back* side of the body. This begins to make sense when you consider that all the activities we do in life take place in front of our bodies. We are constantly reaching forward (driving, typing, reading, cooking), stepping forward (walking, going up stairs, getting in and out of things) and looking forward, which means that we are constantly contracting the muscles in the front side of the body. When muscles contract they become shorter, and if they aren't stretched back to their original length then eventually the shortness becomes the new normal. Over time, this turns into slouching shoulders, forward head carriage, and a rounded upper back. In other words, Upper Cross Syndrome. The stretches in this flexibility routine will focus on combating poor posture by lengthening the front side of the body. I've also included some hamstring stretches because this is yet another muscle group that is prone to tightness.

One more benefit of good posture: it makes you look taller and thinner. If you've ever read an article in a fitness magazine that talks about how you can "lose 5 pounds instantly by standing up straighter", well, it's true. Do your stretches!

Core Strength is the third component of your fitness plan. Core strength is to the fitness world what gluten free is to the diet world: everyone's talking about it but no one seems to truly understand what it is. By definition, the core consists of all the muscles that are attached to the lumbo-pelvic-hip complex, thoracic spine, and cervical spine. In a nutshell, it's all the muscles that encircle your ribs, back, and waist. As it turns out, there are no fewer than 29 muscles included in the core, the majority of which do *not* fall into the sub-category of abdominal muscles. And all this time you thought that core was just another word for abs!

Muscles of the Core:

- Transverse abdominus
- Internal and external obliques
- Multifidi
- Lumbar transversospinalis
- Rectus abdominus
- Erector spinae
- Quadratus lumborum
- Adductor complex
- Quadriceps
- Hamstrings
- Gluteus maximus

That's right, the gluteus maximus (your butt!) is part of your core. Why? Because it helps stabilize and move the lumbo-pelvic-hip complex, which is the skeletal (bones) part of your core. In fact, all the muscles of the core help to stabilize your torso in one way or another, which is why core strength is a big player in maintaining correct posture. If your core muscles aren't strong enough to hold up the bones in your torso, then you will be more prone to slouching and slumping. So now you can start to see how flexibility and strength are related: Poor flexibility leads to poor posture, and so does lack of strength. That's why I've chosen to focus on the strength and function of the core in this workout program as opposed to more "traditional" strength training exercises like biceps curls and leg presses.

Based on the explanation above, you might say that the exercises in the Core Strength section are practical, or "functional". Functional strength training is a type of exercise that has gained increasing popularity in the last 10 years, and for good reason. By definition, functional strength training focuses on exercises that mimic movements we perform in our everyday lives, or the "function" of how we live. This type of training recognizes that the human body moves through space, and that it requires a high level of balance, stability, and strength in order to perform optimally. After all, doing countless sets of seated biceps curls on a machine is fine for creating pretty beach muscles, but it doesn't do much to help you reach into the back seat and grab that 30 pound bag of groceries. Functional strength training involves movements that are multi-planar (moving in several different directions), multi-joint (moving more than one muscle group at a time), and work to improve neuromuscular efficiency. If this all sounds complicated, don't worry - the Core Strength section comes with detailed descriptions and pictures to help you achieve a tight, sexy, functional mid-section.

Phase I Workout Schedule

Focus:

To burn calories through moderate cardiovascular exercise, to improve flexibility through regular stretching, and to build strength and tone the core musculature.

Workout breakdown:

*Four Cardio workouts totaling 130 minutes
*Two Flexibility routines totaling 10 minutes
*Two Core Strength routines totaling 20 minutes

Total weekly workout time: 2 hours, 40 minutes

	Type of Exercise	Duration	RPE
Monday	Cardio of your choice	30 minutes	6
	Flexibility routine	5 minutes	3-4
Tuesday	Rest Day*		
Wednesday	Cardio of your choice	30 minutes	5
	Core Strength routine	10 minutes	5-6
Thursday	Cardio of your choice	40 minutes	6
	Flexibility routine	5 minutes	3-4
Friday	Rest Day*		
Saturday	Cardio of your choice	30 minutes	5
	Core Strength routine	10 minutes	5-6
Sunday	Rest Day*		

*I encourage you to do the Phase I Flexibility routine on your rest days.

Phase II Workout Schedule

Focus:

To increase the endurance and intensity of your cardiovascular workouts, to continue addressing tight and restricted muscle groups through flexibility routines, and to give additional challenges to the core musculature through variation in your strength routine.

Workout breakdown:

*Four Cardio workouts totaling 155 minutes
*Three Flexibility routines totaling 15 minutes
*Three Core Strength routines totaling 30 minutes

Total weekly workout time: 3 hours, 20 minutes

	Type of Exercise	Duration	RPE
Monday	Cardio of your choice	30 minutes	7-8
	Flexibility routine	5 minutes	4-5
Tuesday	Rest Day*		
Wednesday	Cardio of your choice	45 minutes	6
	Core Strength routine	10 minutes	6-7
Thursday	Flexibility routine (do it twice)	10 minutes	4-5
Friday	Cardio of your choice	45 minutes	6
	Core Strength routine	10 minutes	6-7
Saturday	Rest Day*		
Sunday	Cardio of your choice	35 minutes	7-8
	Core Strength routine	10 minutes	6-7

*I encourage you to do the Phase II Flexibility routine on your rest days.

Phase III Workout Schedule

Focus:

To maximize caloric burn through cardio interval training workouts, to create functional flexibility through an active stretching routine, and to create full body strength and stabilization through an advanced core strength routine.

Workout breakdown:

*Five Cardio workouts totaling 185 minutes
*Three Flexibility routines totaling 25 minutes
*Three Core Strength routines totaling 30 minutes

Total weekly workout time: 4 hours

	Type of Exercise	Duration	RPE
Monday	Cardio interval routine	25 minutes	7-9
	Flexibility routine	5 minutes	4-5
Tuesday	Cardio of your choice	45 minutes	6
	Core Strength routine	10 minutes	6-7
Wednesday	Flexibility routine (do it three times)	15 minutes	4-5
Thursday	Cardio of your choice	45 minutes	6
	Core Strength routine	10 minutes	6-7
Friday	Cardio interval routine	25 minutes	7-9
	Flexibility routine	5 minutes	4-5
Saturday	Rest Day*		
Sunday	Cardio of your choice	45 minutes	6
	Core Strength routine	10 minutes	6-7

*I encourage you to do the Phase III Flexibility routine on your rest day.

Exercise Log

(Make copies of this page and fill one out each day)

Date:_____

Day on GF Fat Loss Plan:_____

Type of Exercise	Duration recommended	Duration completed	Quality of workout
Flexibility			
Cardio			
Strength			

Total exercise time today:_____

Total exercise time this week:_____

Jane's Gluten Free Fat Loss Story

I started on the Gluten Free Fat Loss Plan in January, 2010. I'm one of those people who never really knew what gluten was, and I've never exhibited symptoms of having gluten intolerance or being allergic to gluten or wheat. However, once Allison explained how it could facilitate losing weight off my mid-section, I decided to jump in with both feet. I didn't have a lot to lose, but I also felt like I had never reached my true physical potential. After trying numerous diets and cleanses and never losing the weight around my belly, I figured that going gluten free was worth a shot. Wow, what a difference it made! Within a month I had lost 10 pounds, and it all came off my stomach and hips. I went from a size 29 jeans to a size 27, and I've kept it off for almost a year now.

People have asked me if it was hard to cut gluten out of my diet when technically I didn't have to for medical reasons. I stopped eating gluten cold turkey and did not miss it at all. My body acclimated very quickly to a gluten-free diet and I immediately felt benefits such as weight loss, increase in energy and endurance, and sharper mental perception. It is well worth giving up gluten for the amazing benefits your body will feel!

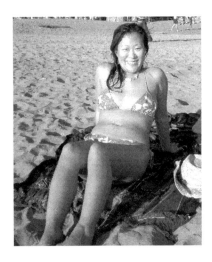

Jane Before

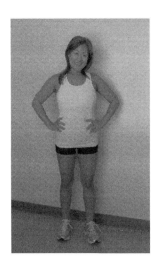

Jane After

Chapter 8

Exercise Demonstrations and Photos

Flexibility Routine Phase I

Exercise #1:

Standing chest stretch in doorway/corner of room

Muscles stretched:

Chest, Shoulders
(Pectoralis major, Pectoralis minor, Anterior deltoid)

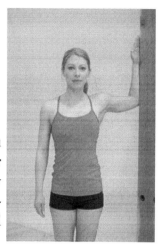

Directions:

Stand tall with your chest lifted, knees soft, and tailbone tucked. You can do this stretch one arm at a time as demonstrated in the picture, or you can put both arms up if you're using a corner of the room. Gently move your elbow up and down the doorway until you find the position that creates the deepest stretch in the front of your shoulder and chest.

Hold for 30 seconds minimum on each arm.

Exercise #2: Floor quadriceps stretch

Muscles stretched:

Front of legs from hips down to knees
(Quadriceps, Psoas, Hip flexors)

Directions:

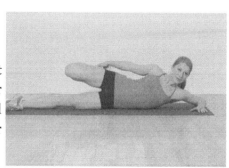

Lie on your left side on a mat or carpet with your left arm extended overhead for balance. Reach back with your right hand and capture the top of your right foot. Keeping your knees as close together as possible, gently begin to pull your right heel toward your right glute as you tuck your tailbone.

Hold for 30 seconds minimum on each side.

Exercise #3: Anterior deltoid/SCM stretch

Muscles stretched:

Shoulders, Neck
(Anterior deltoid, Sternoclidomastoid (SCM)

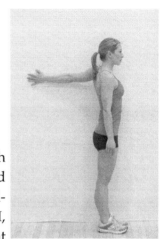

Directions:

Standing next to a wall, reach your left hand behind your body with palm facing the wall and thumb pointed up. Gently lift your chest and pull your right shoulder and hip further to the right. Relax your shoulder blades away from your ears. To get a deeper stretch in the SCM, tilt your head backwards and slightly to the left as if you're looking at something in the left corner of the ceiling. Repeat stretch on the right side.

Hold for 30 seconds minimum on each arm.

Exercise #4: Static lunge stretch

Muscles stretched:

Front of legs from hips down to knees
(Quadriceps, Hip flexors, Psoas)

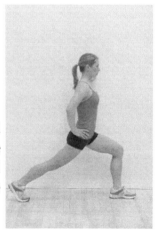

Directions:

On a mat or carpet, place left foot on the ground in front of you and extend right leg out behind. Pull shoulder blades back and make sure upper body is perpendicular to the ground. Tuck tailbone under and gently begin to shift your hips forward until you feel a stretch in the front of your right leg. Switch legs.

Hold for 30 seconds minimum each leg.

Flexibility Routine Phase II
Exercise #1: Upward facing dog stretch

Muscles stretched:

Chest, Front of shoulders, Abdominals
(Pectoralis major, Pectoralis minor, Anterior deltoid, Rectus abdominus)

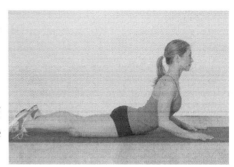

Directions:

Lie face down on a mat or carpet. Slightly press the tops of your feet and hips into the ground. Place your hands directly below your shoulders and squeeze your shoulder blades down and back while squeezing your elbows toward each other. Look down at the mat so that the back of your neck is long and slowly begin to lift your chest off the mat. Try to keep your neck relaxed and as little weight as possible in your hands.

Hold for 30 seconds minimum.

Exercise #2: Standing quadriceps stretch

Muscles stretched:

Front of legs from hips down to knees
(Quadriceps, Hip flexors, Psoas)

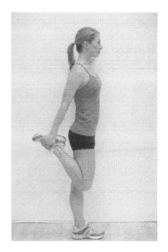

Directions:

Stand next to a wall, chair or table for support. Keeping your tailbone tucked and your knees as close together as possible, gently pull your right heel toward your right glute. Lift your chest and gently push your hips forward a few inches while pulling up on your right foot with your right hand.

Hold for 30 seconds minimum on each leg.

Exercise #3: Supine hamstring stretch

Muscles stretched:
Back of legs
(Hamstring complex:Semitendinosus, Semimembranosus,
Biceps femorus)

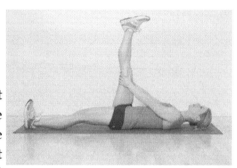

Directions:
Lie supine (face up) on a mat or carpet with both legs extended straight out on the ground. Gently press your left heel into the ground while lifting your right leg toward the ceiling. Try to keep your right leg as straight as possible and grab behind the thigh, knee, or calf to pull your right leg closer to your chest. Relax your shoulders, face and feet.

Repeat on the other leg.

Hold for 30 seconds minimum on each leg.

Exercise #4: Figure four stretch

Muscles stretched:
Outer hip and buttock
(Gluteus medius, Gluteus minimus, Tensor facia latae,
Piriformis, Iliotibial band)

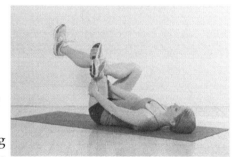

Directions:
Lie supine on a mat or carpet with both legs extended out straight on the ground. Bend your right leg and place your right ankle on top of the left knee while you begin to pull your left leg toward your chest. Reach behind the left leg and gently pull the leg in while you push the right knee out to the side. Repeat on the other side.

Hold for 30 seconds minimum on each leg.

Flexibility Routine Phase III
Exercise #1: Moving hamstring "T" stretch

Muscles stretched:
Outer hip, Buttock
(Hamstring complex, Iliotibial band, Gluteus medius, Piriformis, Quadratus lumbar)

Directions:
Lying supine on a mat or carpet, extend your left leg straight along the ground and your right leg straight up in the air.

Gently pull the right leg in toward your chest, then release your grip and allow the right leg to swing across the body to the left toward the floor. Return right leg to upright position and then lower down to the ground. Lift left leg and repeat.

Do 5-10 repetitions on each leg.

Exercise #2: Prone scorpions

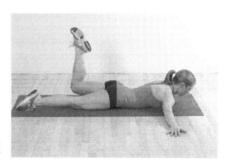

Muscles stretched:
Front of legs from hips down to knees
(Quadriceps, Hip flexors, Psoas)

Directions:

Lie prone on a mat or carpet with your right leg straight and arms out in a T position.

Bend the left leg and lift and straight up toward the ceiling, then twist from your torso and place the left toe on the ground about 12" outside of the right hip. Return the left leg to the ground and repeat with the right leg, creating a rocking sensation from side to side.

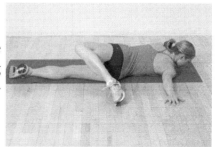

Do 5-10 repetitions on each leg.

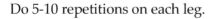

Exercise #3: Prone shoulder/chest stretch

Muscles stretched:

Chest, Front of shoulders, Neck
(Pectoralis major, Pectoralis minor, Anterior deltoid, SCM)

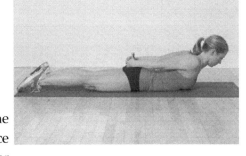

Directions:

Lie prone (face down) on a mat or carpet. Gently press the tops of your feet and your hips into the mat and interlace your hands behind your back. Squeeze your shoulder blades down and together at the same time that you're pushing your hands further down your back towards your heels. Begin to lift your chest off the mat and give an extra squeeze in your shoulder blades. Hold at the top of the movement for 1-2 seconds then relax back down to the mat.

Do 5-10 repetitions of lifts.

Exercise #4: Static lunge to hamstring stretch

Muscles stretched:

Front and back of legs from hips down to knee
(Quadriceps, Hamstrings, Hip flexors)

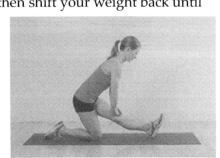

Directions:

Begin in a lunge position on a carpet or mat with your left leg forward and right leg back. Keep your upper body perpendicular to the ground, tailbone tucked and shoulder blades squeezed together. Gently press your hips forward to increase the stretch in the front of the right leg and hold for 1-2 seconds, then shift your weight back until you are almost sitting on your right heel.

The left leg should now be straight with your left toes pointing up to the ceiling. Slowly tilt your upper body forward over your left leg to increase the stretch in the left hamstring. Return to starting position of lunge with the left leg forward and right leg back.

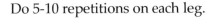

Do 5-10 repetitions on each leg.

Core Strength Routine Phase I
Exercise #1: Opposite arm/leg reach

Muscles worked:
Core muscles, Hips, Shoulders, Entire back
(All of the core muscles listed on page 89, Anterior deltoid)

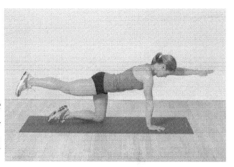

Directions:
Get onto your hands and knees on a carpet or mat. Be sure hands are directly under hips and knees. Pull your belly button slightly in and up and begin to lift your left hand and right foot off the ground at the same time.

Keep your hips and shoulders parallel to the ground and squeeze the right glute to keep the right leg straight. Reach the fingers and toes in opposite directions and hold for 2 seconds. Bring the left hand and right knee back down to the mat at the same time. Repeat on the other side.

Do 2 sets of 10 repetitions on each side; rest for 45 seconds between sets.

Exercise #2: Plank hold

Muscles worked:
Core muscles, Shoulders, Hips
(All of the core muscles listed on page 89, Anterior deltoid)

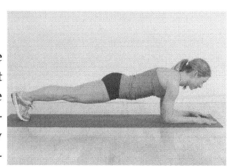

Directions:
Get onto your elbows and toes on a carpet or mat. Be sure that elbows are directly under your shoulders and that your body is in a straight line from head to toe - don't pike your butt up to the ceiling or let your lower back sway toward the ground. Pull your bellybutton in and up, gently squeeze your shoulder blades toward each other and continue to breathe deeply.

Do 2 sets of this exercise, holding each plank for as long as possible; rest for 45 seconds between sets.

Exercise #3: Basic squat

Muscles worked:

Front and back of legs front top of hip down to the ankles, Core muscles for stabilization

(Quadriceps, Glutes, Hamstrings, Core musculature, Calf muscles)

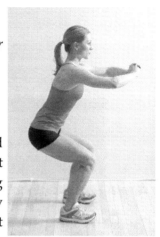

Directions:

The squat is one of the most-used movements in life (getting in and out of a chair, a car, the toilet…) so you need to really work on correct form. Stand tall with your weight in your Heels - try slightly picking your toes up inside your shoes. With your hands on your hips, slowly begin to sit back as if you were reaching for an invisible chair. Do not let your knees come past your toes and do not let your chest drop down toward the ground. Don't be scared to really push your butt back and get the weight in your heels. You can even try this with a chair behind you at first to act as a safety net. Squeeze your glutes and return to starting position.

Do 2 sets of 10 repetitions; rest for 45 seconds between sets.

Exercise #4: Hamstring bridge

Muscles worked:

Back side of the body from the mid-back down to the knees
(Hamstrings, Glutes, Low back)

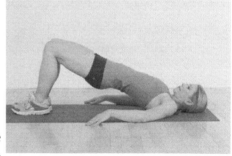

Directions:

Lie on your back on a carpet or mat. Place your feet on the ground approximately 6"-8" from your glutes and keep your knees directly over your ankles. Squeeze your glutes and begin to lift your back off the ground at the same time you're tucking the tailbone. Work to keep the knees hip distance apart and continue squeezing your glutes. Hold at the top for 5 seconds then slowly lower back down to the ground.

Do 2 sets of 10 repetitions; rest for 45 seconds between sets.

Core Strength Routine Phase II

Exercise #1: Opposite arm/leg reach with ab crunch

Muscles worked:

Core muscles, Hip complex, Shoulders, Entire back
(All of the core muscles listed on page 89, Anterior deltoid)

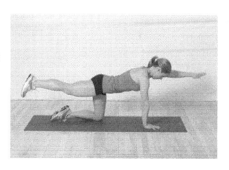

Directions:

Get onto your hands and knees on a carpet or mat. Extend the left hand out straight in front and right leg straight behind. Curl your back up toward the ceiling like a cat and draw your left elbow in to touch your right knee. Concentrate on lifting your bellybutton as high as you can and contracting your abs.

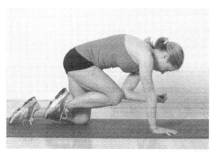

Do 2 sets of 10 repetitions on each side; rest for 30 seconds between sets.

Exercise #2: Plank hold with side toe taps

Muscles worked:

Core muscles, Hip complex, Shoulders
(All of the core muscles listed on page 89, emphasis on Gluteus medius and Tensor fascia latae in the hips, Anterior deltoid)

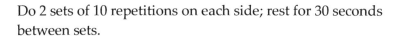

Directions:

Again we see an exercise from Phase I except now with more of a strength and stability challenge. Get into a plank hold on a carpet or mat, keeping the elbows directly under the shoulders and the body in a straight line from head to heels.

Gently pull your bellybutton in and up, pick up your right foot and tap it out to the side approximately 12"-16" from the body. Without rocking your hips, return the foot to starting position and repeat on the left side. Continue to alternate feet while keeping the hips, back, and shoulders still.

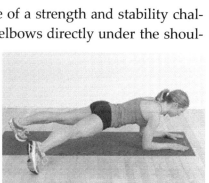

Do 2 sets of 10 repetitions on each foot; rest for 30 seconds between sets.

Exercise #3: Basic squat with arms overhead

Muscles worked:

Almost the entire body!

(All of the core muscles listed on page 89, Quadriceps, Glutes, Hamstrings, Calf muscles, Shoulders, Back muscles)

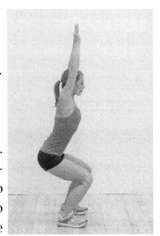

Directions:

Stand tall and pull your shoulder blades together and down your back. Slightly tuck your tailbone and raise your arms straight overhead, being careful not to bend the elbows or let the hands fall foreward to where you can see them. Keeping your weight in your heels, begin to push your hips back as if sitting in a chair. Don't let the knees come past the toes or the chest drop forward toward the floor. Keep the arms overhead and rise back up to standing.

Do 2 sets of 10 repetitions; rest for 30 seconds between sets.

Exercise #4: Hamstring bridge with knee lifts

Muscles worked:

Back side of the body from the mid-back down to the knees
(Hamstrings, Glutes, Low back)

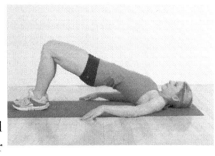

Directions:

Lie on your back on a carpet or mat. Place your feet on the ground approximately 6"-8" inches from your glutes and keep your knees directly over your ankles. Squeeze your glutes and begin to lift your low back off the ground at the same time you're tucking the tailbone. Work to keep the knees hip distance apart and continue squeezing your glutes.

From this position, carefully lift your right knee toward the ceiling approximately 4"-6" inches. Keep the hips level the entire time. Gently set your right foot down on the ground and repeat on the left side, continuing to alternate legs until you reach 10 reps on each leg.

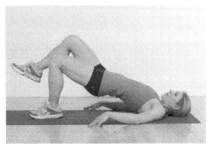

Do 2 sets of 10 repetitions on each leg; rest for 30 seconds between sets.

Core Strength Routine Phase III

Exercise #1: Opposite arm/leg reach on toes

Muscles worked:

Core muscles, Hip complex, Shoulders, Entire back
(All of the core muscles listed on page 89, Anterior deltoid)

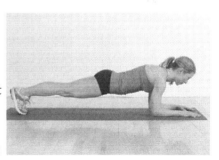

Directions:

Begin in a push-up position on a carpet or mat. Be sure to keep the hands directly beneath the shoulders, stay up on the toes, and create a straight line from your head to your heels. Gently pull your bellybutton in and up, squeeze your glutes and begin to lift your left hand and right foot off the ground at the same time.

You did this exercise on your knees in Phase I, and now it's time to really challenge your balance and strength! Extend as far forward as possible through the left fingers and as far back as possible through the right toes. Don't let the right hip turn up toward the ceiling or the left shoulder collapse toward the ground. Return the hand and foot to the ground at the same time and switch sides.

Do 3 sets of 10 repetitions on each side; rest for 30 seconds between sets.

Exercise #2: Plank hold walk-up

Core muscles, Hips, Shoulders, Entire back
(All of the core muscles listed on page 89, Anterior deltoid)

Directions:

From a plank hold position, shift your weight into your left forearm and place your right hand on the ground.

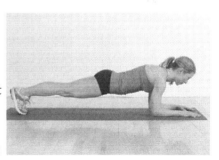

Now shift the weight into your right hand and place your left hand on the ground so that you end in a push-up position.

Reverse the movement to get back to your original plank hold, placing your right forearm down on the ground first, then the left forearm. The goal is to keep the hips as steady as possible during this movement so that the core is forced to stabilize the entire body. Do 5 repetitions leading with the left hand, then 5 leading with the right hand.

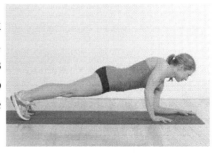

Do 3 sets of 5 repetitions on each side (10 total walk-ups per set); rest for 30 seconds between sets.

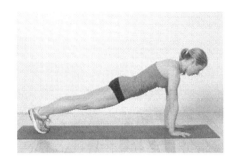

Exercise #3: Single leg squat

Muscles worked:

Front and back of legs front top of hip down to the ankles, Core muscles for stabilization

(Quadriceps, Glutes - emphasis on gluteus medius, Hamstrings, Core musculature, Calf muscles)

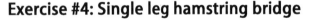

Directions:

From a standing position, place your hands on your hips and lift your left foot 6"-8" off the floor. Utilizing the same good squat form described in Phase I, begin to slowly lower down.

It is extremely difficult to achieve the same depth with a single leg squat as you can with a double leg squat, so be sure to stop as soon as you feel your upper body leaning forward and/or your knee moving forward over your toe. Do 10 repetitions then switch to the other leg.

Do 3 sets of 10 repetitions on each leg; rest for 30 seconds between sets.

Exercise #4: Single leg hamstring bridge

Muscles worked:

Back side of the body from the mid-back down to the knees (Hamstrings, Glutes, Low back)

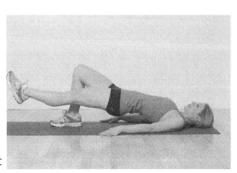

Directions:

From your bridge position, extend your left leg out straight and parallel to the ground. Keeping both hips level, lower down and tap your left heel on the ground. Squeeze your glutes and raise your left leg back up until you reach the top of your bridge. Do 10 repetitions on your left leg, then switch and do 10 on the right.

Do 3 sets of 10 repetitions on each leg; rest for 30 seconds between sets.

What to do if an exercise is too difficult

Don't worry if you find yourself ready for Phase III of the workout program, yet can't seem to conquer those stubborn Single Leg Squats. You can substitute the same exercise number in the previous Phase until you feel ready to try the more challenging exercise again. For example, you can do all the exercises from the Phase III Core Strength program except #3: Single Let Squats. Instead, just do #3 from Phase II. And don't forget to keep track of your workouts with the exercise log provided on page 94.

Chapter 9

Creating Your Own
Gluten Free Fat Loss Success Story

Buying a book that outlines how to lose weight and get fit won't do you any good if you read it, then proceed to let it collect dust on the shelf. If you have actually read all the way through this book and find yourself here, at Chapter 9, then you can give yourself a huge pat on the back because you've not only decided that you want to shed those pounds and get in shape, you've also made the commitment to educate yourself about how to do it effectively. The Gluten Free Fat Loss Plan is not a short-term diet: it's a lifestyle, it's a way to take control of how you nourish your body, and most importantly it's an answer to your weight loss struggles. For good.

I want you to be the next Gluten Free Fat Loss Success Story. So before you start this program, I want you to get some baseline numbers. You'll never be able to see how far you've come if you don't know where you started. I want you to take a before picture (that means NOW!) and place it in the space on the next page labeled "Before". Take another picture when you reach Phase II, and a final one when you reach Phase III, because this means you've hit your goal weight. I made the mistake of not taking official "before" pictures of the four people who are featured in this book as success stories, so I had to ask each of them to dig through their shoeboxes to find me something to use. This was a much harder task than I anticipated. Each of them brought me pictures that showed them half hidden behind other people, holding objects in front of themselves, or drowning in figure-hiding clothes. One of them explained this to me by pointing out that "when you're fat, you don't want anyone having photographic evidence of it."

I respect that you may not want pictures out in the public domain, but the pictures I'm asking you to take are for you and you alone. Use your "before" photo as motivation when you're having a day (week?) when you're tempted to throw in the towel. Look at that photo, close your eyes, and re-commit to living a healthy, lean, gluten-free lifestyle. In a short time you'll be able to open your eyes and look with pride at a photo from Phase II, and shortly after that you'll be gazing at that 8x10 you have framed of yourself that shows off your gorgeous Phase III body!

In addition to taking pictures, I'm going to ask you to keep track of weekly measurements and weight. Sometimes the number on the scale will stubbornly stick, but the measurements will show progress, or vice versa. This is why it's important to keep track of both.

Good luck to you on this incredible journey. If you're in need of some additional support, some new recipe ideas, or want to connect with other people who are living a Gluten Free Fat Loss life, then please visit our online community at www.glutenfreefatlossplan.com, or come say hi on our Facebook page. Welcome to your new life of gluten-free-dom!

Your Gluten Free Fat Loss Success Photos

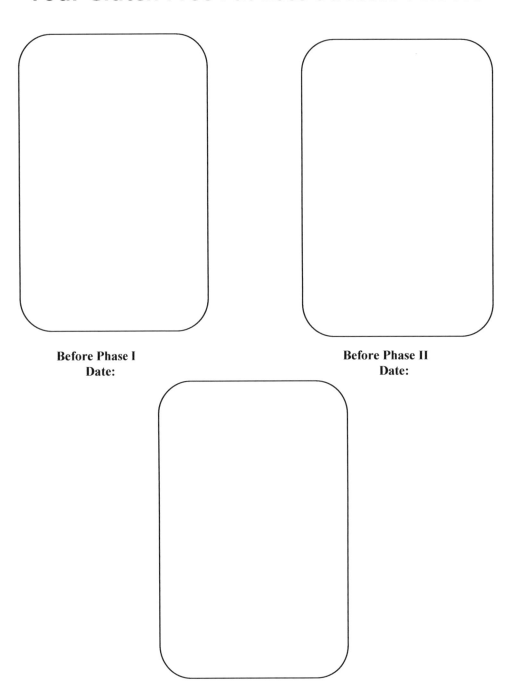

Before Phase I
Date:

Before Phase II
Date:

Phase III - I did it!
Date:

Weekly Measurements and Weight

Take your starting measurements before you begin the Gluten Free Fat Loss Plan, then take them at the end of each week after that. Explanations of how to take measurements correctly are on the next page.

Date: _____

Weight to nearest 0.1 pound:_____

Body Part	Measurements to nearest 1/8 inch	Change from last week +/-	Change from start of program +/-
Waist			
Hips			
Thigh			
Calf			
Bicep			
Chest (men only)			

Pounds lost this week:_____

Total pounds lost:_____

Body Fat %:_____

Body Fat change this week:_____

Total Body Fat change:_____

Weeks on Gluten Free Fat Loss Plan:_____

How to take body measurements and calculate body fat

To take measurements you will need a flexible measuring tape such as a tailor's or dress-maker's tape. You can purchase one at your local Target-type store. Always do your measurements at the same time of day, preferably first thing in the morning.

- **Waist:** measured directly at the belly button. Be sure tape is even the entire way around the waist and isn't higher or lower in the back.
- **Hip:** measured at the fullest part of the hip. Stand with your feet together and don't contract your glutes.
- **Thigh:** measured on the upper portion of the leg where the circumference is the biggest. Be sure to measure the same leg each week.
- **Calf:** measured at the fullest part of the calf.
- **Bicep:** measured halfway between the top of the shoulder and the elbow. Do not flex.
- **Chest:** measured directly at nipple line. Be sure tape is even the entire way around the torse and isn't higher or lower in the back.

Calculating body fat is much trickier than taking measurements. There are numerous methods for measuring body fat, and all of them come with some significant pros and cons. The current gold standard of body fat measuring is called a DEXA scan, or dual energy X-ray absorptiometry. Sounds expensive, doesn't it? It is. Because a DEXA scan uses X-ray technology to measure both the amount and exact location of your body fat, it comes with a high price tag. You can expect to pay anywhere from $100-$500 for this test. However, you do get a lot in return: a map of your body that shows the exact location of body fat, as well as a break-down of how much fat you have in each leg, each arm, your torso, and your head (yes, we have fat in our heads!). The margin of error for this type of test is about 1%-2%, so you walk away with very reliable results. If you have the time, money, and interest, make the investment in getting a "before" scan. Follow the program for 3-4 months and then get an "after" scan. Watching a tangible image of yourself shrink over time is very satisfying.

A cheaper and more convenient option is going to be a body fat analyzer that uses Bioelectrical Impedance Analysis (BIA). The use of the term "bioelectrical" may seem scary, but these analyzers are completely harmless to the human body. An extremely weak electrical current is sent out through the monitor into the body. The amount of current that returns to the sensor will determine the amount of fat tissue in the body. Because fat tissue has less electric conductivity than muscles, blood vessels, and bones, the analyzer is able to calculate an estimated total body fat percentage based on how much resistance it has to go through in the body. The downfall to these monitors is that it is an estimate. You will enter your height, weight, age, gender, and activity level into the monitor and it will use this information plus the BIA reading to calculate your supposed percentage of body fat. The margin of error on a typical BIA monitor is about 5%, which is not ideal by any means but it does give you a nice ballpark from which to start. There are typically two versions of this product: one that is held in front of the body while squeezing handles, and one that is built into a bodyweight floor scale. You can purchase either of these versions online or at a sporting goods store for as little as $25. I encourage you to do your research and read online reviews before you make a purchase. Sometimes cheap is just cheap, so make sure you aren't wasting your money.

Once you have your BIA monitor or scale, don't get caught up on the day to day (or even hour to hour) fluctuations in the readings, but instead pay attention to the trend of the number over time. If you're getting readings of 25%-28% when you start and two months later the monitor regularly reads 15%-18%, then you know you've made serious progress. In order to reduce the likelihood of incorrect readings, be sure to take your reading at the same time of day each time, and strive for a similar amount of hydration in the body. Remember that BIA analyzers get their readings from measuring conductivity in the body. If you chug 30 ounces of water and step on the scale one day, then step on the next day *after* you've just expelled 30 ounces of sweat during a workout, you're going to get wildly different readings.

At this point you might be wondering why I haven't suggested using calipers to measure your body fat. After 10 years of experimenting with every body fat analyzer, measurer, and high-and low-tech machine on the market, I have landed firmly in the camp of "Anti-caliper." I have two main reasons for this opinion. First, the potential for human error during measurement is quite high. Unless you put a permanent mark on each part of the body that is measured, there is no way to guarantee consistency in the location of the pinch. Second, and most importantly, it's virtually impossible to take caliper readings on your own, which means you must recruit someone else to do it for you. When was the last time you wanted to stand half-naked in front of someone (who, by the way, will inevitably be a fitness professional and therefore in great shape) while they pulled your fat away from your body and pinched it into a vise-like contraption? It's humiliating, it's discouraging, and it's not accurate. Get yourself a body fat scale and take your measurements in the privacy of your own home.

Chapter 10

Frequently Asked Questions

Can I mix and match meals from different days of the meal plan?

Yes and no. You can swap out meals as long as you still follow the allowed amounts of foods from each category. For example, if you are in Phase I (which only allows one fruit from the grey category) then you shouldn't have a Blueberry Banana Muffin for breakfast and then a snack that consists of yogurt and a banana. That's too many bananas in one day. You could, however, have the muffin for breakfast and then have the yogurt with berries for a snack (since the berries aren't a grey category fruit).

What if I miss a meal or snack - should I make it up later?

First of all, never miss a meal or snack! But if this happens, make a judgment call on how you feel after you eat the next prescribed meal. If you missed your morning snack and then get right back on track with your lunch, afternoon snack, and dinner, and you feel satiated after dinner then you're probably ok. If you finish dinner and still feel famished, then you can go ahead and eat your morning snack as an "after dinner" snack so that you don't go to bed hungry. But beware that making a habit out of missing meals and snacks is an excellent way to derail your diet. People who don't eat for extended periods of time (more than 5 hours) have a much greater tendency to overeat at their next meal. I always make sure I have a single serving packet of peanut butter, a piece of fruit, or some nuts in my bag when I leave the house just in case I find myself without time to sit down for a full meal. That way I can be sure to stave off the hunger monsters before they come crashing through the door and make me eat everything in sight!

It's difficult to find gluten-free products in my town - what should I do?

As recently as 10 years ago, gluten-free foods were a class of specialty food items that had to be ordered online or purchased at small, natural food stores. But how the times have changed, and quickly! The *Kroger* grocery store chain has published a "Gluten Store Guide", *Safeway* markets have an in-store brand called "O Organics" that offers dozens of gluten-free choices: heck, even the Amish-owned market in my rural Kansas hometown is now offering gluten-free baking flour. However, if after an exhaustive search of your grocery aisles you still find that the products you want aren't available, you essentially have two options:

1. Stick with the foods that are naturally gluten free and readily available in any market. Fruits, veggies, protein, rice, corn tortillas, and sweet potatoes are just a few examples. The great thing about this diet is that it doesn't *require* you to eat exotic and hard to find foods.

2. If you do decide that you want to explore some of the really fun and yummy gluten-free grains such as buckwheat, quinoa, and almond flour, you can easily order them online. Here are a few websites that will ship almost anywhere in the country:

*www.myglutenfreemarketplace.com (does not ship to Alaska or Hawaii)

*www.udisglutenfree.com (I used Udi's gluten-free bread when figuring the caloric value for the sample meal plans)

*www.glutenfreemall.com

Can't I just cut back a little on gluten?

This is a slippery slope, my friend. If you remember from Chapter 3, gluten foods can trigger cravings and food binges, even in very small amounts. In my experience, once people start to cheat with a cracker here, a small piece of bread there, it's not long before they're completely off the wagon and right back to eating their old gluten-filled diet. Furthermore, if you are one of the many people out there who have a gluten intolerance, you won't experience all the amazing additional health benefits of being completely gluten free (refer back to Chapter 4 for a complete list) if you're intentionally or unintentionally consuming gluten. You see, that's the real bummer about eating gluten - even a small little bite actually has the same effect on your digestive system as eating an entire bowl full. You've already made the decision to try out a gluten-free diet, so be committed and make sure that it's entirely gluten free!

I've been on the diet for two weeks and haven't lost a pound - what's wrong?

Though unusual, I have seen this happen. Again, it's very rare, and 99% of the time it is due to one of the following circumstances:

1. *Not being prepared with your meals and snacks.*

This is hands down the most frequent reason that people don't lose weight. Here is a story I've heard time and again from my clients:

> *I didn't have time to eat breakfast, so I ran out of the house with a cup of coffee and a banana. Then I got stuck in a meeting all morning and didn't have a snack with me, so I waited until lunch. They ordered in lunch for everyone at the meeting and it was pizza and soda, so I had to eat it. After the meeting I had a doctor's appointment that took all afternoon, and I was starving by 4 p.m. so I went to the vending machine and got some pretzels. Then I got home late and I was too tired to go to the grocery store, so I just ate a frozen burrito that I found in the freezer.*

Sound familiar? Days like this happen when you aren't prepared with your meals. It is absolutely critical that you plan out your meals and make sure you set yourself up for success by having these foods available. If you aren't in control of what foods are available to you, it will be impossible to make good choices because you won't have a choice - the food will choose you.

2. *Not drinking enough water.* Dehydration can be a powerful force when it comes to weight loss, or lack thereof. If you are chronically dehydrated, your body won't digest food efficiently, you will feel constantly hungry, and your body won't be able to properly eliminate waste. Those eight little water glasses are on the food tracker chart for a reason-make sure they are all getting ticked off by the end of the day!

3. *Not keeping your food journal.* I said it before and I'll say it again: Studies have shown that people underestimate the number of calories they are eating by as much as 40%. If you don't write down every single item that goes into your mouth, you put yourself at risk of unintentionally over-eating and consequently you won't lose weight. Write. It. Down.

PART THREE

Gluten Free Fat Loss Recipes

Choosing ingredients for the recipes

My focus in these recipes is to provide you with delicious and satisfying gluten-free ideas that are also healthy. To this end, I strongly encourage you to purchase organic, locally-raised ingredients whenever possible. Check out your local farmer's market, natural food store, or better yet - start your own garden! Choosing fresh, organic ingredients will make both your body and your taste buds happy.

I've talked extensively about the importance of whole grains, and I'd like you to use whole grain options whenever possible in these recipes. For example, use whole grain (gluten-free, of course) bread for the sandwiches, whole grain pasta for the noodle dishes, and focus on brown rice instead of white. If you're having a hard time locating whole-grain options in your local stores, be sure to check out the list of on-line stores on page 161 that will ship these items directly to your house.

Abbreviations used in the recipes

tsp= teaspoon
tbsp= tablespoon
oz= ounce

Breakfast

Shakes and Smoothies

Soups/Salads/Sandwiches

Appetizers and Snacks

Vegetables and Side Dishes

Main Courses

Desserts

*These items can be prepared vegan

Breakfast

Blueberry Banana Muffins
Phase I, II, III

1/4 fruit, 1/2 grey category fruit, 1 carbohydrate,1/4 protein, 1/2 fat

The sweetness from the bananas is all that's needed for this delicious breakfast treat. Try cutting them in half and placing them in a toaster oven for a few minutes to get that perfectly crisp top.

3 cups Bob's Red Mill all purpose gluten-free flour
¼ tsp sea salt
1 ½ tsp baking soda
½ tsp cinnamon
2 tbsp grapeseed oil (can substitute olive oil)
½ tsp vanilla
3 large eggs
1 tbsp no sugar added applesauce
2 cups mashed very ripe bananas
1 cup fresh blueberries

Preheat oven to 350°.

Combine the flour, salt, baking soda, and cinnamon in a large bowl and stir until mixed. In a medium sized bowl, combine the grapeseed oil, vanilla, eggs, and applesauce and beat. Add this mixture to the flour mixture and stir with a wooden spoon until combined. Stir in the bananas and blueberries but don't overmix. Spoon the mixture into 12 lined muffin tins and bake for 35 to 40 minutes.

Makes 12 servings, 1 muffin per serving

Per serving: 177 Calories, 4.8g Fat, 5.1g Protein, 32g Carb, 4g Fiber, 7g Sugar

Blueberry Almond Oatmeal
Phase I, II, III

1/2 fruit, 1 carbohydrate, 1 fat

This is a quick, filling breakfast that is a perfect combination of protein, fat, and complex carbs. Be sure to use a brand of oatmeal that is gluten free. I recommend Bob's Red Mill.

½ cup slow cooking oatmeal, dry
1½ cups water
¼ tsp salt
⅛ cup sliced or chopped almonds
¼ cup fresh or frozen blueberries (no sugar added)

Combine the oatmeal, water, and salt in a medium saucepan and bring to a boil. Reduce heat and simmer for 5 to 8 minutes until oatmeal is soft and desired thickness is reached. If you like your oatmeal a little runny, add more water. Remove from heat and immediately stir in the blueberries. Allow to cool for 2 to 3 minutes before sprinkling the almonds on top.

This recipe will keep overnight in the refrigerator. Just add a little water to the refrigerated mixture in the morning and heat it up in the microwave or in a saucepan on the stove. Be sure to cover the oatmeal with a paper towel so it doesn't explode in the microwave!

Makes 1 serving

Per serving: 296 Calories, 11.1g Fat, 10.3g Protein, 40g Carb, 8g Fiber, 5g Sugar

Cheesy Breakfast Tacos
Phase I, II, III

1 fruit, 1/2 grey category protein, 1/2 protein, 1 carbohydrate, 1 other

4 corn tortillas (non-GMO)
1 whole egg, plus 3 whites
1 tsp chili powder
¼ tsp paprika
Salt and pepper to taste
2 oz cheddar flavor rice cheese shreds (can use soy or almond cheese)
4 tbsp no-sugar-added salsa
1 small serving of fruit

Heat a heavy skillet to medium heat. Do not grease it. Place the corn tortillas one at a time (or two if your skillet is big enough) and warm them 1 minute on each side, or until they are soft. Remove tortillas to a plate. Now spray bottom of skillet with olive oil spray and add the whole egg plus egg whites. Add the chili powder, paprika, salt and pepper and scramble the eggs. When the eggs are almost done, add the rice cheese shreds and stir until the cheese melts. Place two tortillas on each plate, and put ¼ of egg mixture in each tortilla, then top with a little bit of salsa. Serve with a side of fruit.

Makes 2 servings, 2 tacos per serving

Per serving: 276 Calories, 6.2g Fat, 13.3g Protein, 39g Carb, 3g Fiber, 8g Sugar

Traditional Farmer's Breakfast
Phase II, III

1 fruit, 1 grey category vegetable, 1 grey category protein

It doesn't get any more down-home than eggs, potatoes, and fresh fruit. If you don't have the patience or inclination for hash browns, you can substitute 2 slices of gluten-free toast.

1 egg
1 serving gluten-free frozen hash browns (be sure to check the ingredients for wheat)
½ cup fresh fruit of your choice

Preheat the oven and prepare the hash browns according to package directions. While the hash browns are cooking, prepare the egg any way you like. Scrambled, over easy, hard boiled. Eater's choice! When the potatoes are done, serve alongside the egg and fruit.

Makes 1 serving

Per serving: 267 Calories, 14.2g Fat, 9.3g Protein, 29g Carb, 3g Fiber, 6g Sugar

Spinach and Mushroom Scramble with Gluten-free Toast and Jam
Phase III

2 vegetables, 1 protein, 1 grey category protein, 1/2 grey category carbohydrate, 1 other

1 whole egg plus 2 egg whites
1 cup fresh spinach, chopped
¼ cup mushrooms, sliced
1 tsp Italian seasoning
1 slice gluten-free bread, toasted (*Udi's Whole Grain Sandwich Bread* is used for nutritional calculation)
1 tbsp *Smucker's* low sugar strawberry jam (do not use the sugar-free version, which has artificial sweeteners in it)

Lightly spray skillet with olive oil cooking spray and heat to medium. Add the eggs and cook for 2 minutes, stirring often. Add the spinach, mushrooms, and Italian seasoning and cook for another 2 to 3 minutes or until eggs are completely cooked. Serve with toasted gluten-free bread and low sugar jam.

Makes 1 serving

Per serving: 241 Calories, 8g Fat, 19g Protein, 23g Carb, 3g Fiber, 8g Sugar

Shakes and Smoothies

Breakfast Smoothie
Phase I, II, III

1 fruit, 1 protein, 1/2 fat, 1-1/2 other

What better way to start your day than with a delicious, creamy breakfast smoothie that's packed with quality protein and antioxidants? The key to making this smoothie über -healthy is to use a high quality protein powder. I recommend Jay Robb's brand. Use either whey, egg white, or soy protein. Be sure that whichever brand you buy is free of added sugar, has the word "isolate" after the protein source, is non-GMO, and doesn't contain fake sweeteners.

1 scoop whey protein (whichever flavor you prefer)
½ cup frozen or fresh berries (any combination of strawberries, blueberries, blackberries, etc)
½ cup unsweetened almond milk
1 tbsp almond or peanut butter
½ cup ice cold water
4 or 5 ice cubes as desired

Place all ingredients in a blender or food processor and purée. You may want to add more ice cubes if you prefer a thicker smoothie.

Makes 1 serving

Per serving: 256 Calories, 10.6g Fat, 29.3g Protein, 12g Carb, 4g Fiber, 4g Sugar

Get-Yer-Veggies Smoothie
Phase I, II, III

1 fruit, 1 grey category fruit, 3 vegetables

This smoothie may be green in color, but the banana overwhelms any bitterness that may arise from the veggies. Feel free to add in any other veggies you may have in your fridge: tomatoes, peppers, broccoli, etc. Be creative!

2 cups raw spinach, washed
1 cup any other veggie (except grey category vegetables)
1 medium banana
Handful of blueberries, washed
1 cup ice water

Throw all the ingredients in a blender or food processor and hit puree. I like to pour the smoothie over ice, but feel free to experiment until you find your perfect veggie smoothie.

Makes 2 servings, approximately 1½ cups per serving

Per serving: 70 Calories, 0.5g Fat, 1.8g Protein, 17g Carb, 3g Fiber, 8g Sugar

Post-Workout Recovery Shake
Phase III

1 fruit, 1 1/2 protein, 1/2 fat, 1/2 other

I love this shake after a long cardio day. The combination of protein, fat, electrolytes and antioxidants helps to minimize muscle soreness the next day.

1 scoop vanilla or chocolate whey protein (I recommend *Jay Robb's* brand)
½ cup unsweetened almond milk (*Blue Diamond* makes a good one)
½ cup non-fat greek yogurt (*Fage* or *Oikos* brand)
½ cup frozen strawberries, unsweetened
1 tbsp all natural peanut or almond butter (*Justin's Nut Butter* is fantastic)
1 small scoop *Hammer* electrolyte powder (available at www.hammernutrition.com)
4 ice cubes

Place all ingredients in a blender and blend until you get the desired thickness. If you prefer your shake on the runny side, add a little water. If you like it thicker, add one ice cube at a time until desired thickness is achieved.

Makes 1 serving

Per serving: 336 Calories, 9.6g Fat, 44.3g Protein, 18 g Carb, 4g Fiber, 10g Sugar

Pre-Workout Shake
Phase III

1 fruit, 1/2 grey category fruit, 1/2 fat, 1/2 other

This shake is perfect about 45 to 60 minutes before a workout. It provides glycogen that will be utilized during your workout, and it isn't loaded with refined sugars like most sports drinks.

½ medium banana
½ cup fresh or frozen blueberries
½ cup unsweetened almond milk
½ cup ice cold water
1 tbsp almond butter (*Justin's Nut Butter* is so yummy)
4 or 5 ice cubes if desired

Place all ingredients in a blender and blend until smooth. Consume 45-60 minutes before a workout.

Makes 1 serving

Per serving: 245 Calories, 13.2g Fat, 5.6g Protein, 32g Carb, 7g Fiber, 19g Sugar

Soups/Salads/Sandwiches

African Sweet Potato Stew with Raisins
Phase I, II, III

2 vegetables, 1 grey category vegetable, 1/2 protein, 1-1/2 carbohydrate, 1 other

Recipe submitted by Caroline Blecher and Nancy Beighley, Boulder, CO

1 tbsp olive or grape seed oil
2 cups onion, sliced
2 cloves garlic, minced
1 pound sweet potatoes, peeled and cut into ¼ inch slices
1 large tomato, coarsely chopped
½ cup raisins
½ tsp ground cinnamon
½ tsp crushed red pepper
1 (10.5 oz) can vegetable broth
½ cup water
1 (15 oz) can chickpeas or garbanzo beans, rinsed and drained
4 cups spinach or kale, coarsely chopped
1 cup peas or string beans, either fresh or frozen
4 ½ cups cooked quinoa

Heat oil in skillet and add the onion and garlic. Cook until onion is tender. Now add the potatoes and tomatoes and cook another 5 minutes. Add the raisins, cinnamon, red pepper, peas, broth, and water. Heat this mixture to a boil, then reduce heat to low, cover and simmer 15 to 20 minutes. Add the chickpeas and spinach/kale and cook another 5 minutes or until the chickpeas are heated through. For each serving, spoon 1 ½ cups of stew over ³/4 cup cooked quinoa.

Makes 6 servings

Nutritional information includes ³/4 cup cooked quinoa
Per serving: 332 Calories, 6.4g Fat, 14.4g Protein, 58 g Carb, 11g Fiber, 8g Sugar

Game Day Black Bean Burgers
Phase I, II, III

1/2 grey category vegetable, 1 carbohydrate, 1 other

These burgers are a hit with vegans and carnivores alike. I knew I had struck gold with this recipe when my husband requested I make them for a guys-only football party he was attending.

1 cup black beans, cooked and drained
1 cup garbanzo beans, cooked and drained
¼ cup applesauce (can sub 2 egg whites if desired)
1 tbsp olive oil
1 tbsp wheat-free soy or tamari sauce
1 tbsp dried thyme
1 tbsp fresh parsley
¼ cup grated carrots
2 cups cooked brown rice
salt and pepper to taste

Mix first 8 ingredients in a blender or food processor until a chunky paste is formed. Scoop the mixture out into a large bowl and stir in the rice with a wooden spoon. Add salt and pepper. Form burger-sized patties and place them (I scoop them directly into the pan with a spoon) in a greased skillet. Cook for 4 to 5 min on each side. Add a slice of rice cheese to each burger during the final 30 seconds, then remove from skillet and put it on a toasted gluten-free bun and you have perfection. I like to add sautéed onions and mushrooms and a dollop of guacamole.

Makes 8 servings, 1 burger per serving

Nutritional info does not include bun or toppings added to burger
Per burger: 100 Calories, 2.3g Fat, 3.6g Protein, 17g Carb, 3g Fiber, 1g Sugar

Apple, Chicken, and Goat Cheese Salad
Phase II, III

2 vegetables, 1/2 grey category fruit, 1 protein, 1 fat, 1 other

½ tbsp olive oil
2 (4 oz each) skinless chicken breast
Salt and pepper to taste
4 cups mixed greens
1 Granny Smith apple, unpeeled and cut into small chunks
2 oz goat cheese
2 tbsp walnuts, finely chopped

Heat olive oil in a skillet. Add the chicken breast and cook for 6 to 8 minutes per side, or until the center is no longer pink. Sprinkle the chicken breasts with salt and pepper while it's cooking. Meanwhile, assemble the rest of the salad ingredients in a large bowl. Remove the chicken breasts from heat when it's done, cut into 1" chunks and add it to the top of the salad. Serve with 2 tablespoons vinaigrette dressing of your choice - just make sure it doesn't have any added sugar!

Makes 2 servings

Nutritional info includes 2 tbsp low fat Raspberry Vinaigrette dressing per serving
Per serving: 318 Calories, 16.2g Fat, 32.3g Protein, 14g Carb, 3g Fiber, 8g Sugar

Grilled Turkey Sandwich with Cream Cheese, Sprouts, and Cucumbers
Phase III

1 vegetable, 1 protein, 1 grey category carbohydrate, 1 other

Hooray! Eating gluten free doesn't mean giving up bread or sandwiches. It just means switching to gluten-free varieties.

2 slices gluten-free sandwich bread
3 oz organic roasted turkey breast (must be nitrate free)
2 tbsp dairy-free cream cheese
¼ cup alfalfa sprouts (optional)
4 or 5 slices cucumber (optional)
1 or 2 slices fresh tomato (optional)

Assemble all ingredients into a sandwich. If you feel like using different veggies, go ahead and get creative. I personally love the combo of the crunchy cucumbers and the soft tomatoes. You can easily turn this into a grilled sandwich by popping it into a sandwich grilling machine for a few minutes (i.e. George Foreman grill) or simply grilling the entire sandwich for 2-3 minutes per side in a heavy bottom skillet (if you do this, be sure not to add oil or butter to the sandwich or skillet).

Makes 1 serving

Per serving: 297 Calories, 9.6g Fat, 22.5g Protein, 26g Carb, 1g Fiber, 4g Sugar

Appetizers

Tofu Spring Rolls with Peanut Sauce
Phase I, II, III

1 vegetable, 1/2 grey category vegetable, 1/2 protein, 1/2 other

I love these spring rolls because they take seconds to make, they refrigerate well, and they're a perfect snack food that's healthy and filling.

4 round rice papers (available in specialty markets, or at amazon.com)
1 cup chopped spinach, mixed greens, or combo of both
¼ cup grated carrot
4 oz extra firm organic tofu, sliced into French-fry like strips
4 tbsp chopped fresh cilantro
2 tbsp gluten-free peanut sauce for dipping (I recommend San-J brand)

Dunk individual rice paper in a pie pan full of warm water one at a time. This will make the rice paper soft and pliable. Lay the softened rice paper on a clean countertop or large plate. Place ¼ cup spinach, 1 tbsp carrot, 1 slice tofu, and 1 tbsp cilantro in the center of the paper. Roll the rice paper up like a burrito and seal the edges with your fingers. Place completed spring roll seam side down in a large container or plate. Repeat this process with the remaining 3 rice papers.

Refrigerate completed spring rolls for 30 minutes to chill the rice paper. Serve with a side of gluten-free peanut sauce for dipping.
Try doubling the recipe if you want to have some leftovers.

Makes 2 servings, 2 spring rolls per serving

Nutritional info includes 1 tbsp peanut dipping sauce per serving
Per serving: 56 Calories, 1.8g Fat, 3.4g Protein, 8g Carb, 0g Fiber, 2g Sugar

Crispy Potato Slices with Warm Salmon, Cream Cheese, and Baked Pear
Phase I, I, III

1 grey category vegetable, 1/4 grey category fruit, 1/4 grey category protein, 1/2 fat, 1/2 other

I fell in love with a version of this appetizer that is served at the marvelous Corner Bar in Boulder, CO. I immediately went home to create my own…this is the result.

3 Yukon gold potatoes, cut into ½ " thick slices
2 tbsp extra virgin olive oil
Salt and pepper to taste
1 tsp paprika
½ tsp cayenne pepper
4 tbsp Tofutti cream cheese (can use a different brand)
4 oz smoked salmon, cut into 1" x 1" pieces
1 medium Bosc pear
2 tbsp cilantro, finely chopped

Preheat oven to 350°.

Cut the pear in half and remove the seeds. Place both halves cut side up on a cookie sheet. Place potato slices in a large bowl and add the olive oil, salt and pepper, paprika, and cayenne. Toss until potato slices are thoroughly coated. Lay the slices out on the same cookie sheet as the pear. Bake in oven for 25 to 30 minutes, turning the potato slices halfway through when they begin to brown. Do not turn the pear.

Remove cookie sheet from oven. Place a small dollop of cream cheese on each potato slice, then stack a salmon piece on top of each cream cheese dollop. Return the cookie sheet to the oven for another 7 minutes to allow the cream cheese to warm up and the pear to continue baking. Remove from oven, and carefully slice the pear very thinly lengthwise. Place one thin slice on top of the salmon on each potato, then top if off with a sprinkle of cilantro. Serve the potato slices piping hot!

Makes 4 servings, 3 potato slices per serving
Per serving: 191 Calories, 8.7g Fat, 7.2g Protein, 21g Carb, 2g Fiber, 5g Sugar

Finger Sandwiches with
Roasted Red Pepper Hummus and Cucumber
Phase I, II, III

1 vegetable, 1/2 grey category carbohydrate, 1 other

Small sandwiches are not only a hit at parties, but they are easy to take along to work for a snack. This variation on a common theme is not only gluten-free and dairy-free, but low calorie and healthy! The hummus/cucumber combo gives it a lovely creamy yet crunchy feel.

6 slices gluten-free bread
1 medium cucumber, cut into ¼" slices
³/4 cup roasted red pepper hummus

Lay out 3 of the bread slices on a platter or dish. Spread ¼ cup hummus on each slice, then top with 4 to 5 slices of cucumber. Use the 3 remaining bread slices to complete each of the sandwiches. Cut each sandwich crosswise once, then turn and cut each triangle crosswise again so that you end up with 4 triangle sandwiches from each complete sandwich. This will make 12 small triangle sandwiches.

Makes 6 servings, 2 triangles per serving

Per serving: 127 Calories, 5.1g Fat, 2.8g Protein, 18g Carb, 2g Fiber, 3g Sugar

Roasted Eggplant Roll-ups with Sundried Tomatoes, Goat Cheese and Basil
Phase II, III

1 vegetable, 1/2 fat, 1 other

This recipe is the result of countless hours spent in the kitchen during the summer of '08 with my creative and entertaining sidekick Dani. Thanks for the culinary joy, Dani!

1 medium eggplant, cut into ½" slices
2 tbsp olive oil
1 clove garlic, finely chopped
Salt and pepper to taste
4 oz goat cheese
30 julienne cut sundried tomatoes (get the kind that is not packed in oil)
10 fresh basil leaves

Preheat oven to 350°.

Toss the eggplant, olive oil, garlic, salt and pepper in a large bowl until eggplant is well-coated.

Arrange the eggplant slices on a greased cookie sheet. Do not overlap the slices. Bake for 10 minutes. Remove pan from oven, place a small dollop of goat cheese, 2 pieces of sundried tomato, and one fresh basil leaf on each slice of eggplant. Return to the oven and bake an additional 5 to 7 minutes or until the skin of the eggplant is nicely browned.

Remove from oven, roll each slice up (carefully! They will be hot), and place a toothpick through the roll-up to hold it in place.

Makes 4 servings, 4 roll-ups per serving

Per serving: 175 Calories, 9.2g Fat, 7.5g Protein, 19g Carb, 10g Fiber, 9g Sugar

Gluten-Free Meatballs

Phase III

1/2 grey category vegetable, 1 grey category protein, 1/2 grey category carbohydrate, 1 other

This recipe is printed with permission from the Gluten Free Goddess. You can find more of her amazing recipes at www.glutenfreegoddess.com.

1 small to medium sweet onion
4-5 cloves garlic, peeled, cut in half
1 medium carrot, peeled, cut into several pieces
1 pound of organic grass fed ground beef or buffalo - either works
1 pound of organic ground pork
½ cup Annie's Naturals or Muir Glen Organic Ketchup
1 tbsp organic molasses (this helps bind the mixture)
1 tbsp balsamic vinegar
¼ cup finely chopped fresh Italian parsley
$^1/_3$ to ½ cup gluten-free herbed bread crumbs
¼ tsp cinnamon (the secret ingredient!)
1 tsp fine sea salt
Dash of red pepper flakes, for heat, if desired
Olive oil, as needed

Preheat oven to 350°.
Line a baking sheet with parchment paper. Toss the onion, garlic and carrot pieces into a food processor · and pulse until the texture is very finely diced. Set aside.

In a large mixing bowl, briefly stir together the ground beef and pork. Add in the processed onion, garlic and carrot mixture, ketchup, molasses, balsamic vinegar, parsley, gluten-free bread crumbs, sea salt and pepper flakes. Mix gently to combine. Try not to over-mix (over-mixing makes a dense meatball).

Rub a little olive oil on your hands and form the meatball mixture into balls (golf ball sized). Place them on the lined baking sheet. You should end up with about 20 to 24 balls. Bake the meatballs in the center of the preheated oven for about 30 minutes until done (no longer pink in the center).

Makes 12 servings, 2 meatballs per serving
Per serving: 167 Calories, 5.5g Fat, 20g Protein, 9g Carb, <1g Fiber, 5g Sugar

Vegetables and Side Dishes

Allison's Secret Hummus
Phase I, II, III

1 other

This variation on a traditional hummus has a bit of a kick to it. If you prefer your hummus with a more neutral taste, simply leave out the cayenne pepper.

1 can (10 oz) chickpeas, drained and rinsed, but reserve ½ cup juice from chickpeas
$\frac{1}{3}$ cup tahini
2 tbsp fresh lemon juice
2 tbsp olive oil
$\frac{1}{8}$ tsp black pepper
$\frac{1}{8}$ tsp sea salt
$\frac{1}{8}$ tsp cinnamon
¼ tsp cayenne pepper
2 cloves minced garlic

Put all ingredients (including that ½ cup juice you reserved from the chickpeas) in a blender or food processor and blend until a creamy texture is reached. You can play with the ingredients a bit to suit your taste. For example, you may like more garlic and less tahini, or more cayenne (spicy!) and less cinnamon. Have fun and be creative!

Makes approximately 30 servings, 2 tbsp per serving

Per serving: 38 Calories, 3g Fat, 1.1g Protein, 2g Carb, 1g Fiber, 0g Sugar

Roasted Brussels Sprouts with Medjool Dates
Phase II, III

2 vegetables, 1 grey category fruit, 1 other

Lots of people don't like Brussels sprouts because they can taste metallic, but in this recipe the acidity of the lemon juice and the sweetness of the dates negate any potential icky taste; only roasted yumminess remains!

4 cups Brussels sprouts, washed and cut in half
1 tbsp fresh lemon juice
1 tbsp olive oil
¼ tsp sea salt
⅛ tsp black pepper
3 medjool dates, pitted and finely chopped

Preheat oven to 400°.

Place the Brussels sprouts, lemon juice, olive oil, salt and pepper in a large bowl and toss. Spread the sprouts out evenly in a 9"x 13" glass baking dish. Sprinkle the chopped dates on top. Cook for 10 minutes, toss the sprouts with a spatula, and cook another 10 minutes or until the outside leaves of the Brussels sprouts begin to brown.

Makes 4 servings, number of Brussels sprouts per serving varies depending on size

Per serving: 118 Calories, 3.7g Fat, 3.3g Protein, 22g Carb, 5g Fiber, 14g Sugar

Crispy Polenta Cakes with Sundried Tomatoes and Kale

Phase II, III

2 vegetables, 1-1/2 carbohydrate, 1 fat

The combo of the bitter kale, sweet tomatoes, and crispy corn in this recipe creates an unexpected flavor, and by unexpected I mean excellent!

1 tube pre-made polenta, cut into 8 slices
1 tbsp olive oil
1 clove garlic, finely chopped
4 cups kale, stemmed and loosely torn
½ cup mushrooms, sliced (optional)
10 oil-packed sundried tomatoes, chopped (must be packed in oil)
Salt and pepper to taste

Heat the olive oil in a skillet over medium heat. Place the polenta slices in the skillet and cook 3 to 4 minutes on each side, or until they are crispy and golden brown.

Heat a separate skillet to medium. Add the sundried tomatoes and garlic, being sure to spoon in a little of the oil from the tomato jar. Sauté for 2 to 3 minutes, then add the mushrooms, kale, salt and pepper. Sauté the mixture an additional 3 to 4 minutes to allow the kale to wilt.

Place two slices of the polenta on a plate and scoop ¼ of the kale mixture on top.

Makes 4 servings, 2 slices polenta plus ½ cup topping in each serving

Per serving: 200 Calories, 7.7g Fat, 6.3g Protein, 28g Carb, 5g Fiber, 3g Sugar

Baked Butternut Squash with Apples and Walnuts
Phase II, III

1/2 grey category fruit, 1 vegetable, 1/2 fat

I serve this recipe to guests when I'm trying to convince them that eating gluten-free can still be delicious. It works every time!

4 cups butternut squash, peeled and cut into 1" cubes
2 medium Granny Smith apples, peeled and coarsely chopped
¾ cup white onion, chopped
¼ cup walnuts, finely chopped
3 tbsp olive oil
1 tsp cinnamon
½ tsp sea salt
¼ tsp black pepper

Preheat oven to 350°.

Combine all ingredients in a 9"x 13" glass baking dish and toss until well blended. Bake for 50 to 60 minutes, stirring the dish at 20 and 40 minutes.

Makes 10 servings, ¾ cup per serving

Per serving: 130 Calories, 8.1g Fat, 1.9g Protein, 15g Carb, 2g Fiber, 6g Sugar

Broccoli Quinoa
Phase III

2 vegetables, 1/2 protein, 1-1/2 fat, 2 other

A client of mine raved about a version of this recipe she found online. The original one contains lots of cheese and heavy cream, so I created this healthier variation and it's still just as delicious!

3 cups quinoa, cooked
5 cups raw broccoli, cut into small florets and stems
2 cloves garlic
$2/3$ cup sliced almonds
$1/3$ cup mozzarella style non-dairy cheese shreds
$1/8$ tsp sea salt
2 tbsp fresh lemon juice
3 tbsp olive oil
¼ cup low fat coconut milk

Cook the quinoa according to the package directions and set it aside.
Bring a small amount of water to a simmer in a large pot, then add the salt and broccoli florets and stems. Cover and cook for 1 minute. Immediately remove from heat, strain, and run under cold water so the broccoli stops cooking.
In a food processor or blender, combine 2 cups of the cooked broccoli, the garlic, ½ cup almonds, mozzarella cheese, salt, and lemon juice. Begin to pulse this mixture and add in the olive oil and coconut milk between pulses. Continue pulsing until the mixture is smooth like a pesto.
Now combine the cooked quinoa with ½ cup of the broccoli pesto you just made. Add in the remaining broccoli florets that weren't used in the pesto. You can play with the amount of broccoli pesto you add, as well as the salt and pepper. Serve this with a drizzle of olive oil and a slice or two of avocado on top.

Makes 6 servings, $3/4$ cup quinoa broccoli mixture per serving

Nutritional info does not include added toppings
Per serving: 272 Calories, 16.8g Fat, 7.6g Protein, 26g Carb, 5g Fiber, 2g Sugar

Main Dishes

Baked Halibut with Strawberry Cilantro Salsa
Phase I, II, III

1 vegetable, 1/2 fruit, 1 protein, 1 fat

4 (4 oz each) fresh halibut steaks
1 tbsp olive oil
1 tbsp fresh lemon juice
1 tsp sea salt
1 tsp black pepper
2 tomatoes, chopped
Juice from half a lime
½ avocado, diced
½ red onion, diced
6 strawberries, chopped
1 tbsp cilantro, finely chopped
½ tsp cayenne pepper
1 tbsp olive oil

Combine the first 4 ingredients in a glass dish, cover, and allow to marinate in the refrigerator for at least 30 minutes.

Once you are ready to start cooking, preheat oven to 450°. While the oven is heating, combine the remaining ingredients in a large bowl to create the salsa.

Remove the fish from the refrigerator and set on the counter for 10 minutes to allow the glass dish to come to room temperature. After 10 minutes, place the glass dish (with the marinade still on it) in the oven. Bake for 8 to 12 minutes depending on the thickness of the fish. Remove when fish flakes easily with a fork.

Makes 4 servings, 1 piece of fish and ¼ of salsa per serving

Per serving: 235 Calories, 12.2g Fat, 25g Protein, 9g Carb, 3g Fiber, 3g Sugar

Snow Pea, Pepper and Carrot Stir-fry
with your choice of Shrimp, Chicken, or Tofu
Phase I, II, III

1 vegetable, 1 grey category vegetable, 1 protein, 1/2 fat, 1 other

For the veggies:
1 tbsp sesame oil
1 clove garlic, chopped
1 cup snow peas, washed
1 large red bell pepper, seeded and coarsely chopped
3 medium carrots, peeled and sliced 1/8" thick
1 tsp fresh ginger, finely chopped

For the protein:
1 tbsp sesame oil
12 oz shrimp (peeled, tail off), boneless skinless chicken breast (chopped into 1" pieces) or extra firm tofu (drained and cut into 1" cubes)

For the stir-fry sauce:
1 tbsp cornstarch
4 tbsp wheat-free tamari
2 tbsp rice vinegar
6 tbsp water

For the rice:
Cook 1 cup dry brown rice according to package directions

Begin by getting the rice started. Cook according to package directions (If you don't have a rice cooker, you may want to invest in one. It has personally made my gluten-free cooking a breeze!)

While the rice is cooking, get started with the protein. In a medium skillet or stir-fry pan, heat 1 tbsp sesame oil on medium heat. Add the shrimp, chicken, or tofu and sauté until almost done. The shrimp should be pink on the outside. The chicken should be brown on the outside but still a little pink in the center. The tofu should be golden brown and crispy on all sides. Remove the protein from the skillet and set aside.

Prepare the stir-fry sauce by combining all the sauce ingredients in a small bowl. Whisk until blended and set aside.

Add the other 1 tbsp sesame oil to the skillet and sauté the garlic for 1 minute, stirring often. Add the snow peas, bell pepper, and carrots and cook until they start to soften, approximately 5 minutes. Add the ginger and cook another 2 minutes, continuing to stir. Add in the cooked protein and sauté until the protein is completely cooked, about 1 to 2 minutes. Turn the heat to low and pour in the stir-fry sauce, stirring constantly. The sauce should thicken quickly. Continue to stir for 1 minute until the sauce coats all the veggies and the protein. Remove from heat. Spoon 1 cup stir-fry mixture over rice.*

Makes 4 servings, 1 cup stir-fry mix per serving

Nutritional information does not include rice because the amount of rice you eat with this recipe will vary depending on how many carbohydrates you have left to consume in your day.

Per serving: 197 Calories, 8.1g Fat, 20.8g Protein, 10g Carb, 2g Fiber, 4g Sugar

Spicy Red Pepper and Mushroom Enchiladas
Phase I, II, III

1 vegetable, 1 grey category vegetable, 1 protein, 1 fat, 2 other

1 tbsp extra virgin olive oil
1 clove garlic, minced
½ yellow onion, sliced into rings
2 red bell peppers, sliced lengthwise
10 button mushrooms, thinly sliced
1 tsp chili powder
1 (4 oz) can diced green chilis, medium heat
1 packet taco seasoning mix
10 to 12 corn tortillas (non-GMO)
1 (16 oz) package cheddar flavor non-dairy cheese shreds (rice shreds used to calculate nutritional info)
1 (16 oz) can red enchilada sauce (check for gluten ingredients)
2 tbsp chopped fresh cilantro

Preheat oven to 350°.
Sauté the garlic in olive oil for 2 minutes over medium heat. Add the peppers and onions and sauté an additional 2 to 3 minutes. Add the mushrooms, chili powder, jalapeño, and taco seasoning (with amount of water indicated on back of packet) and sauté until mushrooms are soft and the seasoning mixture begins to thicken.

In a separate skillet, heat the corn tortillas (don't add oil to skillet) for approximately 20 to 30 seconds per side. Remove the tortillas from skillet and put them on a large plate or clean countertop. Place a small amount of the sauté mixture in the middle of each tortilla and roll them up by hand. Spread a very thin layer of the enchilada sauce in the bottom of a 9"x 13" glass baking dish. Place each rolled tortilla seam side down in the dish, pushing them close to each other. Continue to make rows of rolled-up tortillas until the entire baking dish is filled. Pour the remainder of the enchilada sauce over the tortillas. Sprinkle the rice cheese on top. Bake for 30 minutes or until cheese melts and begins to brown slightly.

Remove dish from oven, sprinkle cilantro on top and allow to cool for 10 minutes. Serve enchiladas with dairy free sour cream and guacamole if desired.
Makes 6 servings, 2 enchiladas per serving
Nutritional information does not include sour cream and guacamole
Per serving: 389 Calories, 16.5g Fat, 20.8g Protein, 43g Carb, 5g Fiber, 5g Sugar

Pizza with Fresh Basil, Tomatoes, and Mushrooms
Phase II, III

1 vegetable, 1 grey category protein, 2 fat, 2 other

For the crust:
1 ½ cups almond flour (try *Bob's Red Mill*)
¼ tsp sea salt
¼ tsp baking soda
1 tbsp extra virgin olive oil
1 large egg

For the topping:
¼ cup organic, no-sugar-added pizza sauce
³/₄ cup non-dairy mozzarella flavor cheese (*Daiya* brand used to calculate nutritional info)
2 fresh roma tomatoes (must be very fresh!)
½ cup sliced button mushrooms
10 to 12 fresh basil leaves

Preheat oven to 350°. Prepare the crust by combing the almond flour, sea salt, and baking soda in a medium bowl. In a small bowl, combine the olive oil and egg and whisk together until smooth. Pour the olive oil mixture into the almond flour mixture and stir with a wooden spoon until the mixture forms a firm ball. Place the mixture on a greased pizza pan (or cookie sheet) and press it into a 10" diameter circle using the palms of your hands. If the dough is sticky, flour your hands with a little rice flour.

Spoon the pizza sauce onto the crust and spread it out evenly, leaving a ½" border around the outside of the crust that is not covered with sauce. Sprinkle the non-dairy cheese evenly over the sauce, then place the roma tomato and mushroom slices over the top of the cheese. Bake the pizza for 20 minutes in the oven, then remove it and place the fresh basil leaves evenly on top. Return to oven and bake for another 5 minutes. Remove from the oven and allow to cool 5 minutes before serving.

Makes 2 servings, ½ of the pizza per serving

Per serving: 363 Calories, 25.9g Fat, 7.9g Protein, 19g Carb, 5g Fiber, 4g Sugar

Almond Chicken Cutlets with Peaches and Mangos
Phase III

1/2 fruit, 1/2 grey category fruit, 1 protein, 1 fat, 1 other

3 tbsp fresh lemon juice
2 tbsp agave nectar
2 tbsp olive oil
1 clove chopped garlic
1 tbsp Dijon mustard
2 tsp fresh thyme leaves or ½ tsp dried
$^1/_8$ tsp ground ginger
4 (3 oz each) boneless, skinless chicken breasts
2 fresh peaches, peeled and sliced
1 mango, peeled and sliced
2 tbsp sliced almonds

Preheat oven to 375°. Combine the lemon juice, agave nectar, olive oil, garlic, mustard, thyme, and ginger in a small bowl. Place chicken breasts in a 7"x 11" glass baking dish and coat them with the lemon juice mixture, being sure to cover both sides of the chicken. Arrange the peach and mango slices on top of the chicken, and sprinkle the almonds over the fruit. Bake for 25 minutes, spooning the lemon juice mixture over the chicken every 10 minutes to insure the chicken stays moist. This dish is lovely served over a small bed of brown rice.

Makes 4 servings, 1 chicken breast plus ½ cup fruit mixture per serving

Per serving: 272 Calories, 12.9g Fat, 18g Protein, 23g Carb, 3g Fiber, 20g Sugar

Best-ever Gluten-free Lasagna
Phase III

1 vegetable, 1/2 protein, 1/2 carbohydrate, 1 grey category carbohydrate, 1 other

One package gluten-free lasagna noodles (I strongly recommend *Tinkyada* brand)
One 20-oz jar pre-made organic pasta sauce
1 package non-dairy mozzarella flavor cheese (I use *Daiya* brand)

For the cheese sauce:
¼ cup brown rice flour
¹/₃ cup nutritional yeast
1 tsp salt
2 cups unsweetened almond milk, vanilla flavor
1 ½ tsp cider vinegar

For the dairy-free ricotta:
1 ½ blocks extra-firm tofu
1 tsp agave nectar
2 tsp cider vinegar
1 tsp salt

Preheat oven to 400°.

Cook lasagna noodles in a large stock pot until they are al dente. Remove from heat, strain off water and rinse with cold water. They will continue to cook in the oven once the lasagna is assembled.

While the lasagna is cooking, prepare the cheese sauce and dairy-free ricotta.
Off heat, combine the flour, nutritional yeast, and salt in a small saucepan. Slowly stir in ½ cup of the almond milk with a wooden spoon. Place the saucepan on the stove on medium-low heat, and begin to slowly stir in the remainder of the almond milk and the vinegar. Stir mixture constantly until it begins to thicken and look like a cheesy sauce. Remove from heat.

In a separate bowl, combine all ingredients for the dairy-free ricotta. Crumble the mixture with your hands or a fork until it looks like cottage cheese.

In a 9"x 13" inch glass baking dish, spread a small amount of the pre-made pizza sauce on the bottom. Top with a layer of lasagna noodles, then a layer of the cheese sauce, then more pizza sauce, then a layer of ricotta. Repeat this pattern until all the ingredients are used.

Bake in the oven for 30 minutes. Sprinkle the mozzarella (and fresh basil leaves if desired) on top and return to the oven for another 10-15 minutes or until the cheese starts to bubble.

Let cool for 10 minutes before serving. Enjoy!

Makes 12 servings, each serving approximately 3"x 3" square

Per serving: 272 Calories, 9.2g Fat, 10.8g Protein, 36g Carb, 2g Fiber, 1g Sugar

Desserts

Mom's Homemade Vanilla Lemon Ice Cream
Phase III

Recipe submitted by Margaret Westfahl, gluten free chef extraordinaire (and my mom!)

1/2 cheat food

3 cups unsweetened almond milk
3 egg yolks
1 tbsp arrowroot
$^1/_3$ - ½ cup Grade B maple syrup (depending on how sweet you want)
½ tsp lemon extract (optional)
½ tsp gluten-free vanilla extract

Substitution: $^1/_3$ cup powdered xylitol for the syrup

Beat egg yolks in a blender, then add arrowroot and continue blending. Add milk, syrup and flavorings and blend until well mixed. Pour into 1½ quart size ice cream freezer. I use the type of freezer that doesn't use ice or salt. Freeze for at least 20-30 minutes until the consistency is to your liking.

This ice cream is best if you eat it right away or take it out of the freezer container and put in another bowl and set in your regular freezer for 30 minutes.

Leftovers do not keep well, but you probably won't have any leftovers.

Makes up to 4 servings, ½ cup per serving

Nutritional info uses maple syrup, not xylitol
Per serving: 153 Calories, 5.3g Fat, 2.8g Protein, 24g Carb, 0g Fiber, 20g Sugar

PART FOUR

Appendices, Resources, References

Appendix
Helpful Conversion Charts

Cooking

Unit	Ounces	Dry/Wet conversion
1 tsp	1/6 fluid ounce	1/3 tbsp
1 tbsp	½ fluid ounce	3 tsp
1/8 cup	1 fluid ounce	2 tbsp
¼ cup	2 fluid ounces	4 tbsp
1/3 cup	2 ¾ fluid ounces	¼ cup plus 4 tsp
½ cup	4 fluid ounces	8 tbsp
1 cup	8 fluid ounces	½ pint
1 pint	16 fluid ounces	2 cups
1 quart	32 fluid ounces	2 pints
1 liter	34 fluid ounces	1 quart plus ¼ cup
1 gallon	128 fluid ounces	4 quarts

Common Food Label Measurements

Unit	Conversion
1 gram	0.035 ounces
30 grams	1.06 ounces
50 grams	1.76 ounces
100 grams	3.52 ounces
4.2 grams sugar	1 tsp
1 gram carbohydrate	4 calories
1 gram protein	4 calories
1 gram fat	9 calories

Helpful Websites and Organizations

Foundations and Gluten-free support groups

Celiac Disease Foundation: www.celiac.org
Gluten Free Foundation: www.jackshouse.org
Gluten Free Travel: www.glutenfreetravelsite.com
Gluten Intolerance Group: www.gluten.net
Celiac Disease Center at Columbia University: www.celiacdiseasecenter.columbia.edu
Living Without gluten free magazine: www.livingwithout.com
National Foundation for Celiac Awareness: www.celiaccentral.org
The University of Chicago Celiac Disease Center: www.celiacdisease.net

Recipe Sites

Gluten Free Club: www.glutenfreeclub.com
Gluten Free Easy: www.glutenfreeeasy.com
Gluten Free Goddess: www.glutenfreegoddess.blogspot.com
Gluten Free Gourmet Food: www.glutenfreegourmetfood.com
Gluten Free Help: www.glutenfreehelp.info
Gluten Free Info Web: glutenfreeinfo.com
Gluten Free Mommy: www.glutenfreemommy.com
Glutenfreeda: www.glutenfreeda.com
Gluten.Net: www.gluten.net/recipes/

Online stores
Authentic Foods: www.authenticfoods.com
Gluten Free Mall: www.glutenfreemall.com
Gluten Free Trading Company: www.food4celiacs.com
My Gluten Free Marketplace: www.myglutenfreemarketplace.com
Whole Foods: www.wholefoods.com

Gluten-free Restaurants

This is a list of the major chains that are currently offering gluten-free dishes. For an extensive list of local restaurants, bakeries, caterers, and grocery stores in your area, visit www.glutenfreeregistry.com or www.glutenfreerestaurants.org.

Austin Grill
Biaggi's
Bonefish
Boston Market
Burtons Grill
Carrabbas
Charlie Brown's Steakhouse
Cheeseburger in Paradise
Chili's
Fleming's Steakhouse
Fresh 2 Order
Garlic Jim's
Glory Days Grill
Legal Seafood
Not Your Average Joe's
The Old Spaghetti Factory
Outback Steakhouse
On the Border
P.F. Chang's
Pizza Fusion
Ruby Tuesday
Sam & Louie's
Ted's Montana Grill
Stonewood Grill and Tavern
Uno Chicago Grill
Wahoos Fish Taco
Wildfire

Gluten-free foods by brand names

(I've listed my personal favorite items in parenthesis)

1-2-3 Gluten Free Inc
Allen Creek Farm
Amy's Organics (all of her gluten free frozen meals)
Ancient Harvest
Arica Foods
Blue Diamond (almond nut thins)
Bob's Red Mill (pancake mix)
Chebe Bread (cinnamon rolls)
Deboles
Domata Living Flour, Inc
Elana's Pantry
Ener-G Foods
Enjoy Life Foods
Food Should Taste Good
GFN Foods
Gillian's Foods
Glutenfreeda (frozen burritos)
The Gluten Free Pantry (chocolate brownies)
Hodgson Mills
Kay's Naturals
Kinnikinnick Foods (bagels)
Laura's Wholesome Junk Food
Lundberg (all varieties of risotto)
Mr. Krispers
Mr. Ritt's
Mrs. Leeper's (Beefy Mac Meal)
Namaste Foods
Natasha's Health Nut Cookies
Pamela's Products
Rustic Crust
Shabtai Gourmet
Sweet Baby Cakes
Sweet Street Desserts
Thai Kitchen (peanut sauce, soy sauce)
Tinkyada (all pasta varieties)
Udi's (whole grain sandwich bread)
Vitapath Foods

Glossary of Terms

Bioelectrical Impedance Analysis (BIA)
A method of approximating body fat percentage by running an extremely weak electrical current through the body via a monitor (usually in a floor scale). The amount of current that returns to the sensor on the monitor will determine the amount of fat tissue in the body, as fat has less electric conductivity than muscles, blood vessels, and bones. This information is combined with information entered by the user about height, weight, age, gender, and activity level.

Bran
One of three parts of a kernel of wheat, the bran contains the largest amount of soluble fiber. Bran is removed during milling to make refined, enriched, and bromated flour, but is left intact for the creation of whole grain flour. It can also be bought separately.

Cardio workout
Cardio workouts are any type of activity or sport that elevates the heart rate. Cardio workouts are included in this program as a means of burning calories and increasing cardiac conditioning.

Celiac disease
An autoimmune disorder that results in the complete inability to digest gluten, celiac disease causes damage to the villa in the small intestine and interferes with absorption of nutrients from food. Other terms for celiac disease are celiac sprue, nontropical sprue, and gluten-sensitive enteropathy.

Celiac sprue
See definition for Celiac disease.

Endosperm
The largest part of a kernel of grain, the endosperm constitutes almost 83 percent of kernel's total weight and is the source of white flour. The endosperm contains the greatest share of protein, carbohydrates and iron, as well as the major B-vitamins, such as riboflavin, niacin, and thiamine. It is also a source of soluble fiber.

Enriched grains
Grains that have been refined (bran and germ removed) and stripped of key nutrients such as fiber, iron, and folic acid. After processing, these nutrients are added back in, thereby enriching the grain. Many times the nutrients that are added back are not in the same form; for example, metallic iron can be used. Furthermore, added nutrients commonly represent a fraction of what the original grain contained.

Exorphins
This term was first used by scientists Zioudro, Streaty and Klee in 1979 to describe the opioid- (narcotic) like effect that pieces of milk and wheat proteins (peptides) can have on the human body. Exorphins are also found in gluten protein.

FDA

The Food and Drug Administration, which is funded and run by the United States government. The FDA is responsible for protecting the public health by assuring the safety, efficacy and security of human and veterinary drugs, biological products, medical devices, the United States food supply, cosmetics, and products that emit radiation. For a more complete explanation of the FDA's responsibilities and actions, visit www.fda.gov.

Flexibility workout

Flexibility refers to the relative ability to move joints and muscles through a full (or optimum) range of motion. Lack of flexibility results in decreased range of motion, joint stiffness, and lack of blood flow to soft tissue in the body.

Fortified grains

Essentially the same as enriched grains, except that fortified grains have nutrients added to them that never originally existed in the grain, as opposed to nutrients that once existed but were removed.

Germ

The germ is the embryo or sprouting section of the seed or kernel of weight, and it constitutes about 2 ½ percent of the kernel weight. The germ is removed from flour when making enriched, refined, and fortified flour, but is retained in whole grain flour. The germ contains minimal quantities of high quality protein and a greater share of B-complex vitamins and trace minerals.

Gliadin

Gliadin is a protein found in the endosperm of wheat, barley, and rye. It combines with the protein glutenin to help form gluten.

Gluten

Gluten is a binding protein found in wheat, barley and rye. More specifically, it is two proteins called gliadin and glutenin. These proteins are found in the endosperm of the aforementioned grass-related grains.

Gluten derivative

Foods and food products that are derived (made) from rye, barley, or wheat. Many times these products do not contain the words rye, barley, or wheat. For a complete list of foods that contain gluten derivatives, refer to pages 23-26.

Gluten intolerance

Characterized by distress resulting from eating gluten-containing products. Individuals with gluten intolerance may experience a variety of symptoms ranging from gastrointestinal distress to emotional instability to skin irritation. Unlike with celiac disease, there is no indication that consuming gluten will cause damage to the villi of the small intestine. Other terms for gluten intolerance include gluten sensitivity and non-celiac gluten intolerance.

Gluten sensitive enteropathy
See definition for Celiac disease.

Gluten sensitivity
See definition for Gluten intolerance.

Gluten-free
This is a catch-all term that refers to any food product that is either naturally gluten-free or has had any gluten-containing ingredients removed.

Grey category foods
In The Gluten Free Fat Loss Plan, certain foods have been designated as "Grey category" foods because they are restricted due to their level of sugar, carbohydrates, saturated fat, or all three.

Non-celiac gluten intolerance
See definition for Gluten intolerance.

Nontropical Sprue
See definition for Celiac disease.

Per capita
Per capita is a measurement that refers to the amount of something that is used, consumed, or required per person per year. For example, in the United States, the per capita sugar consumption is 156 pounds, meaning that each person in the United States consumes (on average) 156 pound of sugar per year.

Prone
A position of the body in which the person is face-down.

Rate of perceived exertion
Also referred to as RPE, this is a subjective means of gauging how hard a person is working during a workout, and it is measured on a scale of 1-10 (some literature will use a scale of 1-20).

Refined grains
This type of grain has been modified or refined from its original composition by removing the bran and germ. Refining techniques frequently include mixing, bleaching, and bromating.

Strength workout
A type of resistance-based workout in which strength is increased by performing exercises with added weight (i.e.dumbbells, barbells, and cables), body weight, or both.

Sub-clinical
Sub-clinical is a medical term that refers to a disease or condition that is suspected but not detected. Many people suffer from sub-clinical gluten intolerance.

Supine

A position of the body in which the person is face-up.

Upper Cross Syndrome

Upper Cross Syndrome is a common postural distortion that describes a compromise in the musculoskeletal system. This syndrome is characterized by a tightening of the muscles in the anterior (front) aspect of the upper body, and a weakening of the muscles of the posterior (back) torso. More common terms used for Upper Cross Syndrome are slouching, hunching, and poor posture.

USDA

The United States Department of Agriculture. The USDA is a government-run organization that provides leadership on food, agriculture, natural resources, and related issues based on sound public policy, the best available science, and efficient management. For more information on the USDA, visit www.usda.gov.

Villous atrophy

Villous atrophy is an abnormality of the small intestinal mucosa, which results in a flattening of the mucosa and the appearance of atrophy (weakening) of the villi. People who suffer from celiac disease exhibit villous atrophy.

Whole grains

Whole grains consist of the intact, ground, cracked or flaked caryopsis, whose principal anatomical components - the starchy endosperm, germ and bran - are present in the same relative proportions as they exist in the intact caryopsis. See page 22 for a diagram of a whole kernel of wheat.

Bibliography

Altobelli, Lisa. "A system designed by a Navy SEAL got the Saints' Drew Brees in shape to succeed." *SI.com* January 9, 2007. http://sportsillustrated.cnn.com/2007/players/01/09/nfl.workout0115

Bowden, Jonny. *The 150 Healthiest Foods on Earth.* Massachusetts: Fair Winds Press, 2007: 74.

Case, Shelley. *Gluten free Diet: A Comprehensive Resource Guide.* Revised and expanded. Canada: Case Nutrition Consulting Inc., 2010.

Eberman, Lindsey E., and Michelle A. Cleary. "Celiac Disease in an Elite Female Collegiate Volleyball Athlete: A Case Report." *Journal of Athletic Training* 40(4) 2005: 360-364.

Green, Peter H.R. MD., and Rory Jones. *Celiac Disease: A Hidden Epidemic.* Revised and updated. New York: Harper Collins Publishers, 2010.

Hadithi, Muhammed MD et al., "Accuracy of Serologic Test and HLA-DQ Typing for Diagnosing Celiac Disease." *Annals of Internal Medicine* 147(2007): 294-302.

Hoseney, R. Carl. "*Corn*" from *Principles of Cereal Science and Technology.* St. Paul: 1986.

Howe, Warren B. "Celiac Disease." *Journal of Athletic Training* 40(4) 2005: 370-371.

Huntington, Anna Seaton. "A Debilitating Disease That Is Often Unknown." *The New York Times,* October 10, 2008. http://www.nytimes.com/2008/10/10/sports/othersports/10celiac.html

James, E. Leone et al., "Celiac Disease Symptoms in a Female Collegiate Tennis Player: A Case Report." *Journal of Athletic Training* 40(4) 2005: 365-369.

Lin, B.H., and Steven T. Yen. *The US Grain Consumption Landscape: Who Eats Grain, in What Form, Where, and How Much?* ERR-50. U.S. Dept. of Agriculture, Econ. Res. Serv. November 2007.

Miller, Karen K. "Mechanisms by Which Nutritional Disorders Cause Reduced Bone Mass in Adults." *Journal of Women's Health* 12(2) 2003: 145-150.

Pagano, Amy E. "Whole Grains and the Gluten free Diet," *Practical Gastroenterology* Oct, 2006: 66-78.

Starbucks nutritional information. http://www.starbucks.com/menu/food/bakery/low-fat - raspberry-sunshine-muffin

Stazi, AV., Trecca, A., and B Trinti. "Osteoporosis in celiac disease and in endocrine and reproductive disorders," *World J Gastroenterol* 14(4) (2008):498-505.

U.S. Census Bureau. "Health and Nutrition," *Statistical Abstract of the United States: 2011.* 140.

U.S. Department of Agriculture. "Small Grains 2010 Summary." September, 2010. http://usda.mannlib.cornell.edu/usda/current/SmalGraiSu/SmalGraiSu-09-30-2010.txt

U.S. Department of Agriculture. "Wheat's Role in the U.S. Diet Has Changed Over the Decades." http://www.ers.usda.gov/briefing/wheat/consupmtion/html

U.S. Department of Health and Human Services and U.S. Department of Agriculture. "Dietary Guidelines for Americans, 2005." www.healthierus.gov/dietaryguidelines

U. S. Environmental Protection Agency. "Major Crops Grown in the United States." September 10, 2009. http://www.epa.gov/oecaagct/ag101.cropmajor.html

U.S. Food and Drug Administration. "Food Allergen Labeling and Consumer Protection Act of 2004" (Public Law 108-282, Title II). http://www.fda.gov/food/labelingnutrition/FoodAllergensLabeling/ GuidanceComplianceRegulatoryinformation/UCM179394.pdf

Wangen, Dr. Stephen. *Healthier without Wheat: A New Understanding of Wheat Allergies, Celiac Disease, and Non-Celiac Gluten Intolerance.* Seattle: Innate Health Publishing, 2009: 35.

16643004R00090

Made in the USA
Lexington, KY
04 August 2012